the beautiful balance
balance
for body & soul

the beautiful balance
for body & soul

Cynthia Culp Allen

&

Charity Allen Winters

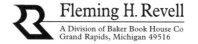

Fleming H. Revell
A Division of Baker Book House Co
Grand Rapids, Michigan 49516

© 2003 by Cynthia Culp Allen and Charity Allen Winters

Published by Fleming H. Revell
a division of Baker Book House Company
P.O. Box 6287, Grand Rapids, MI 49516-6287
www.bakerbooks.com

Printed in the United States of America

Library of Congress Cataloging-in-Publication Data
Allen, Cynthia Culp, 1954–
    The beautiful balance for body and soul / Cynthia Culp Allen and
Charity Allen Winters.
        p.   cm. — (LifeBalance series)
    Includes bibliographical references.
    ISBN 0-8007-5869-2 (pbk.)
    1. Christian women—Religious life. 2. Beauty, Personal. I. Winters, Charity Allen. II. Title. III. Series.
BV4527 .A445 2003
248.8'43—dc21   2003012724

Unless otherwise indicated, Scripture is taken from the NEW AMERICAN STANDARD BIBLE ®. Copyright © The Lockman Foundation 1960, 1962, 1963, 1968, 1971, 1972, 1973, 1975, 1977, 1995. Used by permission.

Scripture marked NIV is taken from the HOLY BIBLE, NEW INTERNATIONAL VERSION®. NIV®. Copyright © 1973, 1978, 1984 by International Bible Society. Used by permission of Zondervan. All rights reserved.

From Charity:

To my mother, Cynthia Culp Allen, and my mother-in-law,
Mary Beth Winters, the two most beautifully balanced women
I know!
And to Kelvin, my beloved, lifelong body-and-soul-mate.

From Cynthia:

To all the beautiful women in my life . . .
my mother and mother-in-love,
my sisters and sisters by marriage,
my grandmothers and great-grandmas,
my aunts and great-aunts,
my girlfriends forever . . .
but especially to my two daughters,
Carly and Charity,

who have taught me far more than I have taught them.

Contents

Acknowledgments

From Charity:

I need to thank two people at the release of this book. First is my new husband, Kelvin Winters, the man who has shown me the reality of unconditional love in a superficial world. He looks at the bare-faced, messy-haired, four-eyed, purple people-eater lying next to him every morning and still seems to think I am the most beautiful woman in the world! (They say "love is blind" and I often find myself thankful for that!) Kelvin, through you I have learned that feeling beautiful comes from knowing you are loved. Thank you for keeping me beautifully balanced in life. You are a gift, and I love you.

And thank you to my mother, Cynthia Culp Allen, the woman who has given me more than any other. She has passed on to me her heart for God and her keen fashion sense. From the temporal to the eternal, she has shared everything with me. Now, Mom, I am also excited to share this journey with you. Thank you for your sacrificial love and the courage to dream. For who you are and who you've helped me become, I am honored to be called your daughter and your friend.

From Cynthia:

There are so many people to thank in the making of a book. My parents, Richard and Geneva Culp, need acknowledgment for building into my life from childhood the foundation of Christ. Thanks for giving me Jesus, Mom and Dad! I love you for it—what a gift!—and I'm eternally grateful.

Thanks to my husband, Charles Allen, for being there through the ups and downs and for providing occasional distractions from my manuscripts. Thanks to my five children for sharing Mom with a computer through the years. They will always be my first priority. I love them more than they will ever know (until they get their own kids, that is!). Charity, Chad, Carly, Caleb, and Christian have encouraged my dream as much as anyone. I hope my success will give them the courage to pursue their God-given dreams without giving up.

I'm thrilled to acknowledge my friends in Colusa, CA, where I began writing this book series. My thanks to Pastor and Penny Scott, Ana and Gonzalo Alvarez, and Sharon and Tony Lopez for all their prayers and support when the giants loomed large upon my entering the Promised Land. Much gratitude goes to my Colusa Bible study class, a Spirit-led group of women who were willing to forego our Precept Bible study "just one time" while I taught these Beautiful Balance principles. Thanks for the fun memories, girls, and God bless you all!

Charity and I have to brag a little about our team at Baker/Revell—the best! Editor Jennifer Leep has been our cheerleader and champion through this multiple-book process, which began as the Body and Soul series and grew into the LifeBalance brand. Jennifer is a joy to work with! Wendy Wetzel has also been a great editor. And we've enjoyed brainstorming and laughing with Cheryl Van Andel (art department) and Twila Bennett (marketing).

Thanks to my two agents at Alive Communications: my former, Linda Glasford, who recognized my talent, and my present, Lee Hough, who has fine-tuned it. (And yes, Linda, wherever you are: I still take bubble baths!)

Charity and I appreciate our business connections with Natren Incorporated and Vitamix International. We are excited about the possibilities that lie ahead for all of us and for the families who will benefit. We have to take a moment to thank Paul Webb, producer at Hollywood Pacific Studios, who has been an exceptional business advisor, friend, and number one fan all along the way. And I can't forget to acknowledge Elaine Wright Colvin, my Christian publishing mentor, who has given advice and provided support through the twists and turns of this particular series.

My special thanks goes to Jesus Christ, for without him, there would be no LifeBalance series. The Beautiful Balance philosophy grew out of years spent in a close relationship with Christ. The series idea took flight as I walked and prayed each day in our almond orchard in Richfield, California, back in 1995. These books have been on a long journey, but each step has been fascinating. Only God knows where the journey will lead, but my prayer is that we touch every person we can along the way!

1

The Beautiful Balance

Beauty is an experience as much as an appearance. If it's true that we are as young as we feel, perhaps it's also true that we are as beautiful as we feel.

How do you view your life today? Do you feel beautiful and balanced, making the most of your assets, ready to use your unique gifts and talents to serve others? Are you a sweet young thing, with a world of blooming possibilities ahead? Perhaps you are a confident middle-ager, secure in life's lessons, satisfied with the present, and hopeful about your future. As an older woman, you may be pleased with your opportunities to share areas of expertise with the younger set, eager to leave your legacy in life.

Or you may be in a slump. Depressed. Unsure. Doubting yourself. Feeling bad about your appearance, regretting some of your choices, not measuring up to what you wish your soul to be. And you just can't muster up the energy or commitment to make the necessary changes in your life. The low self-worth in your heart manifests itself on the surface. This dilemma can happen to any woman at any age.

As a professional model, I (Charity) have had the chance to work with some of the most beautiful young women ever to grace the printed page. Yet the pattern I see remains consistent: The more beautiful the girl on the outside, the more miserable and insecure she is on the inside! Most of these girls are nonbelievers, but the irony of it is still amazing!

I (Cynthia) have been in the beauty business since 1973. I have learned that some women will always think they're too old, too ugly, or too unsuccessful to ever be considered beautiful. They are discouraged, feeling like they'll never find a balance for their lives.

But we've got good news—they are wrong! When a woman learns to emphasize her good qualities, improve areas that can be changed, and finally accept some fixed features, suddenly she feels beautiful, and that radiates to the outside. When a woman begins to care for her body and her soul, she finds balance for her life. These transformations are truly remarkable. And if you are in need of a miracle, it can happen to you!

The first step is in wanting the change enough to work toward it. Wishful thinking gets a person nowhere. But we know you care enough—that's why you grabbed this book off the shelf. You know there is something better for you than the life you're living. You realize that with a little know-how, some extra work, and a firm commitment, you can become all that God intended you to be. The dissatisfaction you feel with your life is just where God has you at the moment; it's the catalyst to bring about his remarkable transformation in your own life. In the following pages, you'll find the advice you need to become the best you can be both inside and out. We will give you tried-and-tested strategies to make the most of your face and figure, along with a creative parallel to your spiritual life—always most important.

You can find a beautiful balance; but first we all need a vision of God's design for us as women.

In the Beginning . . .

Imagine that you are an acclaimed scientist in a state-of-the-art lab. You are about to create the world's most beautiful woman. Where do you start? How will you put her together? Should you give her the classic eyes of Elizabeth Taylor along with Grace Kelly's smile? The statuesque figure of Cindy Crawford might be a nice touch, crowned with the glory of Rapunzel's long, flowing hair. You can use your creative imagination down to her frosted toenails. What fun it would be to view your beautiful finished creation standing before you!

Think of the joy God must have felt when he created the world's first woman, Eve. When he established the earth, he had no model to go by. But when he created man and woman, the Lord had a standard. Not a Hollywood celebrity prototype—even better, he made them in his own image (Gen. 1:26–27). God produced the world *ex nihilo*, out of nothing. He spoke, and it came into being. When creating humankind, the Lord used a medium, the dust of the earth: "Then the LORD God formed man of dust from the ground, and breathed into his nostrils the breath of life; and man became a living being" (Gen. 2:7).

Out of all that God made, the only thing he pronounced "not good" was that man was alone. So God created woman to be a helper suited for Adam. Genesis 2:21–22 tells us that the Lord caused a deep sleep to fall upon the man . . . then he took one of the man's ribs and fashioned a woman from it. The man was formed, but woman was fashioned. (This verse is proof that, from the beginning of time, women have always been fashionable!)

Can you imagine the almighty Creator lovingly, gently fashioning the first woman—molding her curves, coaxing curls into long locks, stroking a blush across velvety cheeks, placing the light in her alluring eyes and an assured smile on lips as smooth as a rose petal? He was preparing a bride for her wedding day. The Lord God brought Eve to Adam, and the man accepted the woman as his own. "This is now bone of my bones and flesh of my flesh; she shall be called Woman, because she was taken out of Man" (Adam's words upon claiming his wife, v. 23). In that glorious garden, the first wedding ceremony was performed. And no one is more lovely than a bride on her wedding day.

Eve was especially magnificent physically, coming directly from the creative hand of God. But she also had that perfect balance of physical and spiritual beauty that every woman desires deep in her heart. God had breathed his life into this first feminine creature. She experienced an unparalleled relationship with her Creator. In addition, Eve enjoyed God-designed intimacy with her husband and lived in harmony with the world around her. Everything was just perfect . . . until she obeyed the voice of the Enemy and her flawless world fell apart.

The Balancing Act

Ever since that time, women have been trying to get back into balance. The ideal is to become a whole person: complete outside, mature inside. But most of the time, it's one extreme or the other. Some women focus on the physical—a beautiful face, body, and home. They put their time, effort, money, attention, and hope into their physical assets. But their spiritual lives are neglected and empty. The world does this because the material, those things we can see and touch and taste and smell, is all the world has.

A Christian woman is privileged to have so much more, both inside and out. Through Jesus Christ, she has been brought back into a kinship with her Creator. Her relationships with others can be restored through the power of the Holy Spirit as she obeys God's Word. Peace and harmony are hers as she lives a life full of love and joy.

And yet Christian women get out of balance too. They can also overemphasize physical appearance. Many times, however, they gravitate to the extreme opposite of the world's perspective. They feel it is more spiritual *not* to pay attention to the physical. They overlook their faces, hair, and bodies, never living up to the potential God placed within them at birth. Mary Crowley, founder of Home Interiors, often said, "God doesn't make no junk." But some of us go around looking pretty trashy week after week. Sometimes even our Christian testimonies are dimmed because of this inconsistency.

The late radio preacher Dr. J. Vernon McGee once shared a letter he'd received from a woman who was turned off by her Christian neighbor. The lady next door constantly pushed McGee's radio broadcast, recommending that the letter writer tune in. But the Christian, who listened to her gospel programs day and night, was a terrible housekeeper, looked a wreck, and had an unhappy husband and five unruly children. The letter ended, "I associated her fanaticism with you, Dr. McGee, and wouldn't listen to your broadcast. Now I listen and get so much out of the study of the Word. I wish I could have seen past that lady's disorderly life a long time ago."

Earlier in life, I (Cynthia) lost opportunities at times because of the way I looked. People were put off by my scroungy appearance, thinking I wasn't sharp, classy, or professional enough for the job. Other times, I lacked confidence in the way I looked (for good reason!) and didn't approach someone as I felt led.

We mustn't let our exterior be a distraction to anyone. First Samuel 16:7 reminds us that God looks on the heart, but people *do* look on the appearance. Remember, we never get a second chance to make a first impression.

Many times, the women of certain philosophical persuasions will all dress a certain way—we can tell what leader they are following by their attire. Some appear to have stepped out of the pages of a history book, circa 1800, directly into the new millennium. In doing so, they defeat the very purpose they are after: not wanting to call attention to the physical. We believe wholeheartedly that God put us into this century, and he intends us to live godly lives here and now. We can dress modestly and still look stylish. It's interesting, too, that most of these people who purposely neglect their physical appearances remodel and redecorate their homes at great expense. We can't understand why, then, it is wrong to polish up the temple of the Holy Spirit. Think of the ornate beauty of the tabernacle and temples of centuries past, as well as the magnificent dress of the priests, according to God's blueprint in Exodus 25–31.

The Old Testament (for example, Genesis 12 and 20) reveals that many of the women of the past were "beautiful," or in the King James, "fair." So beautiful, in fact, that foreign kings kidnapped these fair maidens for their harems. We can't get away from the fact that God designed women to be physically attractive.

Authors Karen Lee-Thorp and Cynthia Hicks offer a balanced perspective in their book *Why Beauty Matters:*

> Our bodies are as much us as our thoughts are. This is why calls to ignore our outer appearance as spiritually irrelevant do not help us. Quite the contrary: the more we honor our

bodies as us, as intertwined with our spirits, as limbs of Christ, temples of the Spirit, and bearers of God's image, the more we will understand and manage well the power of physical appearance in our lives.[1]

Perhaps women who believe that plainness is next to godliness have an interpretation of 1 Peter 3:3–4 that is different from ours: "Your adornment must not be *merely* external—braiding the hair, and wearing gold jewelry, or putting on dresses; but let it be the hidden person of the heart, with the imperishable quality of a gentle and quiet spirit, which is precious in the sight of *God*" (emphasis ours).

These verses, in context, are talking about winning our unbelieving husbands through our godly behavior. The wise counsel is to not *only* be attractive to our husbands physically but to also win them over spiritually with our sweet, Christ-like spirits. If we take these verses out of context, we wouldn't even put clothes on!

Rather, Peter is telling us to nurture our spirits in addition to caring for our bodies. The perfect balance. We are to care for both, recognizing that we are both body and soul. However, the spirit is always more important, "imperishable . . . precious in the sight of God." The majority of our time and attention should focus on our spiritual lives. Our bodies are for this life, but our spirits will live forever.

Honoring God, Body and Soul

We want to be good stewards of all that God has given us: our souls, our faces and bodies, strength and health, time and money, talents, families, homes, and so on. It honors the Lord when we appreciate all his gifts not only in words but also in our caring for our resources.

We know that God cherishes our spirits. He sent his Son Jesus Christ to die for us so we could live eternally. But he also cares about our bodies. According to Matthew 6:28-30, God dresses even the flowers with great consideration.

> "Mark Twain once said, 'God created man because He was disappointed in the monkey.' Well, what purpose does that leave for the creation of woman?"
>
> —Cynthia Culp Allen, twenty-first century philosopher

I (Cynthia) learned this lesson early in life. For most of the summer before entering high school, I worked for some neighbors, taking care of their animals to earn money for school clothes. Growing up in a farm family of eight children (I was the oldest), there was never any money for extras. So I looked forward to spending all of that hard-earned cash on some trendy clothes for my high school debut. But when handed my paycheck, I sensed the Lord telling me that I should send all of it to a certain missionary lady.

"All of it, Lord?" I asked. I could nearly hear his answer: a firm yes.

So I immediately mailed it all off to the widowed missionary with three children, trusting that the Lord would provide what I needed. Within a day or two, my family had a knock on the door. Another neighbor brought over several boxes of clothes that her wealthy niece didn't want. They were just my size, much nicer than I ever would have bought, with the price tags still on. Those clothes outlasted my high school career. And so did the lesson that if we seek God and his kingdom, everything else will be added to us (Matthew 6:33).

Lucille Ball once said, "Love yourself first and everything else falls into line." Well, we disagree with Lucy's philosophy, and so does God's Word. If we make Jesus Christ our number one priority, our first and most precious love, with our full allegiance and commitment going only to him, then, and only then, does everything else fall into line.

Real-life Royalty

A Christlike Christian is wonderful, no matter what she looks like. But a sharp-looking Christian, with godly character and a confident smile, is dynamite! A polished look or professional image, along with that winning smile of yours, can open doors. Others will be drawn to you. When you develop into the beautiful, godly woman that God created you to be—watch out, world! Get excited about all that God can do in and through you. It's not a sin to have some excitement and enthusiasm in one's life. The word *enthusiasm* comes from *en theos,* or "in God." Because we are living securely in Jesus Christ, we can be absolutely giddy over our abundant lives today and our promised glorious future. As we continue to improve inside and out, our families also get really excited, because we represent them. And even more importantly, we represent Jesus Christ.

> "Personal beauty is a greater recommendation than any letter of reference."
>
> —Aristotle, Greek philosopher, 2400 years ago

Princess Diana took seriously her role as representative of the royal family. She always looked the part. Even though we disagreed with her moral standards, we had to respect the way Diana always looked and spoke like a true daughter of royalty. How much more should we present ourselves in that regal style, being daughters of the King of Kings!

Let's look at two women from the Bible who cared about appearances for different reasons. We can use one as our paradigm. This lady found a balance so beautiful that the world still sings her praises. But first, let's talk about our negative example: a woman who loved this world and all that it had to offer more than life itself. Her experience can be our teacher. In fact, Jesus reminded us to learn from her. In Luke 17:32, he said, "Remember Lot's wife."

The Original Material Girl

Lot's nameless wife haunts the Old Testament. Our friend and women's leader Joy Merrill teaches a wonderful class on this poor lady. Joy has given Lot's wife the nickname "Lotus." It's fitting, don't you think? If you know the story, you remember that Abraham had offered his nephew, Lot, the land of his choice. Genesis 13:10–13 says, "Lot lifted up his eyes and saw all the valley of the Jordan, that it was well watered everywhere . . . like the garden of the Lord"—likened to the Garden of Eden, it must have been a beautiful place—"so Lot chose for himself all the valley of the Jordan . . . and moved his tents as far as Sodom. Now the men of Sodom were wicked exceedingly and sinners against the Lord."

Surely, the reputation of Sodom went before it. Who knows why Lot, a man who was later called righteous, chose to move to such a godless place? We can only imagine the influence Lotus might have had on him.

"Lot, honey, what is that you say? Uncle Abraham has offered you the property of your choice? Land of Goshen, Lot! Don't be shy. Take that gorgeous little piece in between those two happening cities, Sodom and Gomorrah. I'm sick of rotting away in this godforsaken desert. I want to live! I was born for glamour and beauty, for culture, for class. Why, with my looks and charm, I could go places. I will be somebody in Sodom, Lot, you'll see. And I won't wait another minute—I'm going to pack!"

Within several years, Lotus's dream had come true. She and her husband had become "somebodies" in the wicked town. Genesis 19:1 says that the two angels, whom God had sent to destroy Sodom and Gomorrah, found Lot sitting at the city gate. It was a place of status; only the "who's who" of that day sat at the city gate. Lotus had arrived, and she was loving every minute of it!

More than likely, her days were spent in beauty treatments at Salon de la Sol: massage and mud baths, hair braiding and hedonism. Lotus's free time also took her to Sodom's Saks and other shops where she freely spent her husband's money, decorating herself and her home. High society parties and events at the country club filled her evenings. Hobnobbing with the rich and famous was what Lotus lived for.

Scripture indicates that there were compromises during the couple's climb to the top. In Genesis 19:7, when the evil Sodomites come to sexually assault God's messengers, Lot pleads with the men, calling them "my brothers." Then Lot offers these perverts his virgin daughters instead. What a dad! The angels explain to Lot that God is about to destroy the evil cities and his family needs to get out. But Lot hesitates (v. 16). The pull of Sodom's world is so strong. Finally, the angels grab Lot's hand, and the hands of his wife and two daughters, dragging them all out of the city to safety. They tell the family to escape for their lives and not to look behind them.

However, as God rains down fire and brimstone, destroying the cities, Lotus looks back. In that instant, she becomes a pillar of salt. A monument to disobedience. A statue foreshadowing the first commandment: "You shall have no other gods before Me" (Exod. 20:3). These are the things Jesus reminded us to learn from her.

We could say, "Gee, that's harsh! Does God have no mercy? One little peek and poof, she's a lump of salt!" But there was so much more in that one little look back. With that backward glance, Lotus was saying, "I don't care what God says. Who does he think he is, anyway? My life is back there, in Sodom. I love those people, those restaurants and stores, my home and possessions. I don't want to leave it all and go on with this God whom I don't even know. I'll worship who or what I want to worship."

If we choose anything over God, we are worshiping that earthly thing instead of our Creator. It could be our looks (or plainness), our home, our fame, our fortune, our family or friends, our education or talents. Our lives are out of balance and our gods enslave us.

Consider this African illustration about how to catch a monkey:

- Step 1: Drop a peanut into a soda bottle and hang it at the top of a tree, along with a net.
- Step 2: Hide in the bushes and wait for a monkey to smell the peanut and come running, or rather, swinging. It won't be long!
- Step 3: Watch as the monkey tries to get the peanut out of the bottle. Suppress your giggles so the monkey won't hear you. He will slip his little hand into the mouth of the bottle. He will pull and pull and pull on that peanut, trying to get it out. But the monkey's clenched fist won't let it. The monkey wants that peanut so much that he can already taste it. The monkey won't let go. You've trapped your monkey!

So often, we are like the poor, unsuspecting monkey in this illustration. We want something so badly that we are willing to risk everything to get it. That thing, feeling, asset, or person is most important to us. We put it or them first in our hearts and lives, to the exclusion of God and his best for us.

Is there anything you are hanging on to today, refusing to let go? Is something keeping you from going on with God? Lotus's life was out of balance. She cared only for physical things—her looks, her possessions, her social circle. She didn't take the time to develop her heart, her inner beauty, which will last for eternity. She had no time for God. And Lotus paid a high price for it.

Lotus wasn't just a b.c. phenomenon, now extinct like the dinosaurs. We are surrounded by Lotuses today. I (Charity) have modeled with girls like this—gorgeous on the outside, shallow and hateful on the inside. If I reach out to them at a photo shoot with a warm smile and friendly word, they never smile back. Instead, they can only offer the "stare down" . . . and often the "glare down"! Some have even met me with a curse. Honestly, it instantly alters your opinion of their beauty.

On the other hand, we may be very much like Lotus ourselves. Cynthia's sister, Sandy, lived next door to a modern-day example of Lotus. We'll call her Velma. Like Lotus, Velma had no time to think about spiritual things. She and her husband were into position and possessions. At forty-two, Velma had recently undergone surgery for a face-lift and tummy tuck. She had just bought over $3,000 worth of new clothes to fit her new figure. Velma owned thousands of dollars' worth of Hummel and David Winter collectibles. She spent lots of money and time on herself and her home.

Don't get us wrong. Velma was a good person. She did lots of volunteer work. And there's nothing bad about buying clothes and collectibles. But Velma took no time to think about spiritual things or to know Jesus Christ. She wasn't interested in going to church or to a ladies' Bible study, to read her Bible or Christian books, or to pray. Velma was too busy to think about the life after this one. Her focus was on the physical and on worldly things. Her life didn't have a biblical balance, and the consequences were serious.

If spiritual topics ever came up, Velma brushed them off, saying, "Some people need God, but I'm not planning on dying." Then one day, Velma and her husband, along with another couple, were leaving in a private plane for a weekend in Las Vegas. She went over to Sandy's house to say good-bye. "We're all packed and ready to go," she said lightheartedly. "See you on Monday."

But Velma never made it home. On the return flight, their plane crashed into the side of a mountain and burst into flames. Everyone and everything inside were burned beyond recognition. The only items investigators found were Velma's wedding ring and a bunch of coins on the floor of the plane, left over from the gambling weekend.

Velma's new face and figure were gone. Her new clothes were left hanging in her closet with the price tags still on. Her collectibles were put into storage "where moth and rust destroy."

Velma wasn't planning on dying. But who really ever is? Velma's life was out of balance. Like Lotus before her, she had emphasized the material without a care about the spiritual. Velma hadn't taken the time to get to know Jesus Christ. And then she was face-to-face with him.

In Revelation 1:17–18, Jesus says, "I am the first and the last, and the living One; and I was dead, and behold, I am alive forevermore, and I have the keys of death and of Hades." In the Book of Revelation, Jesus is revealed as the almighty God and Judge of all the earth. Someday we will all stand before him. When we are weighed on the scale, we want our lives to have eternal weight. Our relationship with Christ should be our top priority, as well as living our lives with an enduring purpose. Scripture is full of women who made a godly impact on their worlds. Let's talk about one of them, a beautiful lady who would make a good mentor for us all.

Another Royal

Princess Diana wasn't the only girl with royal shoes to fill. Persia's Queen Esther (478 B.C.) came from humble beginnings. An orphan of exiled Jews, Hadassah (as she was called) had been raised by her father's nephew, Mordecai. Cousin Morty recognized beauty when he saw it and entered his young charge in the nation's first beauty pageant—a contest intended to win a new bride for the monarch. King Ahasuerus was still brooding over his former wife, Queen Vashti, who had been banished for disobedience.

As soon as the lovely Esther's feet hit the palace floor, she was showered with approval, individual attention, and gifts. Esther 2:9 says that Hegai, the king's eunuch in charge of the contestants, was very pleased with the young woman and she found favor with him. He quickly gave her cosmetics and a special menu, seven of the king's best maids, and the most luxurious apartment in the harem.

For the next twelve months, Esther and the other girls indulged in every kind of beauty treatment. They were oiled and massaged and spiced with everything nice. They spent six months with spices and six months with oil of myrrh. (Forget Oil of Olay—get us some of that Oil of Myrrh; it seemed to work!) The young ladies also learned the fine art of cosmetic application.

When it came time for Esther to go in to the king, she took the advice of Hegai, dressing exactly as he directed. When everyone saw her, they were delighted and showered Esther with favor (Esther 2:15). The king, too, loved Esther, and she found favor and kindness with him more than all the girls, so that he made her queen instead of Vashti (v. 17).

To win the crown, Esther had to find the beautiful balance. She polished up the outside so bright and shiny that she got the king's attention. Then he was compelled to find out what she was like on the inside. And Ahasuerus desired what he discovered: a lovely young woman with a difference—someone even lovelier on the inside.

What if Esther hadn't taken the time to prepare? What if she had gone in to the king with straggly hair, rough skin, and bulging buns, dressed in baggy sweats and a torn T-shirt? The king would have called the guards to throw her out! "What an insult!" he'd fume. He would never have given her another thought. And the godly young woman would have missed the opportunity to serve her Creator in a unique situation.

Instead, Esther made the effort to enhance the physical attributes that God gave her. It paid off with an impact on eternity. However, her adornment wasn't merely external. The king was drawn to the young Jewess by her beauty, but he was captivated by the hidden person of her heart, her sweet, gentle, quiet, peaceful spirit. So unlike the other girls—overly anxious to impress, silly, jabbering nervously, callous, shallow, even empty. The king couldn't wait to get them out of his room. But Esther . . . he wanted to spend the rest of his life with her.

God is a huge part of the love triangle here. The favor that the king and his court continually bestowed on Esther was the Lord's doing. God was working out a plan to use Esther's imperial position to save the Jews from destruction. She was the perfect tool. The wise young queen realized the effectiveness of a beautiful balance. She retained her humble spirit. But she also dressed her finest and looked her best every time she went before the king. When Esther requested something important of her husband, his answer was a resounding yes. How could he say no to this winsome girl, appealing in both body and soul?

Modern-Day Mentors

Jesus encouraged us to remember Lot's wife, never forgetting the consequence of her wrong priorities. But we can all learn from Esther too and even imitate her. The beautiful balance works! When we begin to develop our physical and spiritual selves—without neglecting one or the other—exciting things happen. God used Esther's looks to get her into the place that he needed to fulfill his plan. He can use our attractiveness in the same way for his glory. The Holy Spirit draws people to us so that they come to know the Savior who makes our eyes shine, our smiles warm and genuine, our hearts overflowing with love and joy.

Don't get us wrong. We have no intention of spending a year of our lives devoted to physical appearance. That year was required for Esther's purpose and might be so for beauty queens today. That's why I (Charity) decided not to enter the Miss America and Miss USA pageants when asked to do so. I've had beauty queens as roommates and friends and know firsthand the dedication to physical appearance that they must have. Instead, we want to spend as little time as necessary to look as good as we possibly can. We don't want to waste God's time on the superfluous! And we're sure you don't either. It only takes a few minutes a day to maintain all that he has given us.

All of us have times, however, when we get bogged down in life. We don't take the time we need to be our best. We "fall off the wagon," so to speak, in our grooming and fitness. We stop taking care of ourselves and quit spending time with the Lord. We stop believing that there is anything better for us than what we're experiencing right now. That is not true! It's a lie from the Enemy. God imagined someone beautiful when he created you. No matter what state you're in, no matter how overweight and out of shape; no matter how ignorant of skin care, cosmetics, or Scripture; no matter how young or old; you can begin taking steps to a better and beautiful, more Christlike you.

We can learn how to make the most of our physical attributes while continuing to grow in godliness every day. Through the redemptive work of Jesus Christ, the destruction and division of the fall can be restored to wholeness. The army's slogan, "Be all that you can be," will become our motto as we develop into our complete potential. God has a plan. If we do our part, he will do what only God can do: transform us from the inside out.

We're all in this adventure together. God directs through his Spirit and his Word, and we want to support each other every way we can (see www.lifebalanceladies.com). We know you can do it! However, don't put your life on hold waiting to arrive at the destination (in this case, "the dream you"). In the following chapters, you'll find practical advice and biblical counsel for becoming your best self in body and soul . . . everything you need to reach your goals and enjoy the journey along the way!

2

Makeover Miracles

We live in an age of miracles. Amazing breakthroughs occur in every field of society. Medically, surgeons can operate on an infant still in the mother's womb. And in our technical world, we have voice-activated gadgets such as computers, cell phones, and even cars. Scientifically, we have crossed a monkey and a jellyfish. The poor little primate glows in the dark!

These modern-day "miracles" extend into the beauty and fashion world too. With medical intervention and computer imaging, models flaunt flawless faces and figures. For instance, did you know that for the cover of *Cosmopolitan*, computer pros slimmed down Cindy Crawford's figure in several strategic spots? How would you like to digitize your thighs? Even we common folk can benefit from these advancements. When septuplet mom Bobbi McCaughey's teeth looked less than photo-perfect for a magazine cover, they were technically enhanced, giving her that Hollywood smile.

But you don't need a computer whiz and a studio to be the subject of a makeover miracle. You can create a whole new you in the privacy of your own home. With a little beauty and fashion know-how (provided in the following pages), as well as the life-changing principles of God's Word, you can become a new creation in both body and soul. God has a wonderful plan for you, which includes the person you are becoming and the purpose for which he made you. Remember, you are on an incredible journey. Each step in the direction of your goal—a new you, inside and out—will bring satisfaction to your soul.

Just as it's fun to memorialize a trip or vacation, it's fun and helpful to record the adventure you are about to embark on. Maybe it's the writer in us, but we jot down everything: shopping lists, to-do lists, prayer requests, journalings, lists of goals and dreams, and areas to improve. We have notebooks for writing ideas, others for business, one for Bible study and prayer, and others for our families and households. Sounds like a whole library of notebooks, huh? Why not just use the computer? We both prefer a notebook and pen for that frequent hour when we want to sit by the fire with a cup of tea and plan our lives. Those relaxing times of daydreaming are when the dreams begin to take flight. In addition, these notes keep us on track; we're better able to focus on what we need to do individually to turn fantasies into realities.

The "New You" Notebook

How would you like to be the featured subject of a book? You can be when you write it yourself! For this special subject of inner and outer beauty, you can create a "New You" Notebook—a notebook to hold all the dreams you have for yourself, the goals you want to achieve in body and soul, and the specific steps on how to get there. You will get lots of concepts from this book. And while you are on your journey, ideas will jump out at you from magazines, books, speeches, television, and the Internet. Copy or cut them out and paste them into specific sections in your notebook.

To make your "New You" Notebook, buy an inexpensive loose-leaf binder, the kind that you carried around in high school. Choose your favorite color. Cynthia uses a regular-sized green (to symbolize growth) notebook that holds lined paper (8½-by-11 inches). Charity prefers a smaller, five-by-seven-inch version that travels easier. It can be pulled out of her purse or briefcase quickly when she's waiting at an audition or in church when she's inspired by the pastor's message. A day planner with extra sections and pages can double as a convenient, organized "New You" Notebook. We also like the binders that have the clear vinyl on the front cover so we can display motivational pictures or a personal collage.

Be creative. Use colored pens and markers. Cut and paste pictures and motivational sayings from magazines and newspapers. Save poems that inspire you. Include photos of your own. The book is yours—an expression of who you are and the person you are becoming. You are the celebrity here, so be sure to shine!

Inside its covers, utilize dividers to categorize your notebook however you desire. You can use the subjects from each chapter in this book or come up with your own categories. (If you don't want the work of creating your own notebook, see the appendix for ordering information.) In each section, you might include the following ideas.

Dreams and Goals

In this first section, write down what your personal dreams are. We're thinking "beauty" here, but you can include what-

Cynthia Shares

As a beauty consultant and cosmetologist, I have witnessed many incredible transformations. Right before my eyes, at the touch of my hands, women go from plain Janes to glamour gals. It's always a thrill to see the unique beauty of every client blossom during a makeover session. And no one is more delighted than the woman herself when she looks in the mirror.

ever you want. An example of a physical beauty dream might be this: Your twentieth anniversary is coming up, and you want to go on a cruise with your husband. You plan to look fantastic in a swimsuit! The goals, then, are the steps to make the dream come true. Count how many weeks you have until departure. Plot your weight loss with a detailed diet and exercise plan, as outlined in our companion book, *The Healthy Balance for Body and Soul* (available in early 2004). (You can keep these entries in the Figure section of your notebook.) Research cruise lines on the Internet with your husband; order tickets. Shop for that perfect little swimsuit, and you're good to go!

An example of a spiritual beauty goal might be to become kinder in your dealings with people, more Christlike. You could list verses that you want to memorize in a section in your notebook. Then bring this desire before the Lord in prayer. Record situations where you respond in a godly way, such as when that coworker insults you for the thirteenth time! These are your success stories, and you need to claim your victories in Christ. The dreams that you have for yourself will happen when you put some thought into them and include the Expert in the process.

Have you ever wished for a makeover—physical, spiritual, or both? This is one desire that can come true! It's possible to alter your appearance, to change your body image, and also to be transformed from the inside out. The Bible says that when you receive Christ as your Savior, you are a new creature (2 Cor. 5:17). The old things have passed away. Everything becomes new.

The butterfly has long been a symbol of Christianity and spiritual rebirth. This beautiful creature begins as a humble, brown caterpillar, crawling through life. An innate drive causes it to spin a cocoon for winter hibernation. Thus begins its metamorphosis—a change in form and function—into God's colorful creation made to fly to new heights. Helen Keller once remarked, "One can never consent to creep when one feels an impulse to soar." The Creator made us to aspire to greatness. We want to soar; don't you?

Evaluate Yourself

The first step toward a rising new you, inside and out, begins with self-evaluation. No, you don't have to crawl into a cocoon to do this! And it need not be painful. On the contrary, look at it as an exciting adventure. The future holds an even better you! To be beautiful body and soul, we want to maximize our strengths and minimize (or overcome) our weaknesses. But we have to know our frailties before we can fix them. And fixing them is what we want to do. So ask yourself the following questions, and be very honest as you pencil your answers into your notebook:

- What areas of your physical appearance are you most happy with?
- Is there anything you'd like to change about the way you look?
- Are you healthy and strong, energetic and enjoying life?

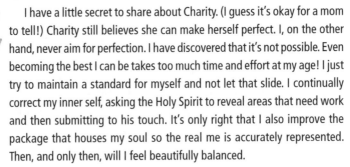

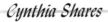

Cynthia Shares

I have a little secret to share about Charity. (I guess it's okay for a mom to tell!) Charity still believes she can make herself perfect. I, on the other hand, never aim for perfection. I have discovered that it's not possible. Even becoming the best I can be takes too much time and effort at my age! I just try to maintain a standard for myself and not let that slide. I continually correct my inner self, asking the Holy Spirit to reveal areas that need work and then submitting to his touch. It's only right that I also improve the package that houses my soul so the real me is accurately represented. Then, and only then, will I feel beautifully balanced.

- What are your personality strengths and weaknesses?
- Write down five words that best describe your physical appearance; then five words that describe your personality.
- Are you able to enjoy loving relationships with family members and close friends?
- Do you feel satisfied with the important areas of your life: home and family, work, friends and social life, church family?
- What about your relationship with God? Is it growing? Do you spend time with him daily, in the Word and in prayer? Is the peace and joy of the Lord your usual experience? Do you have his power to obey Scripture? Are you sharing Christ with others? How do you regularly serve him?

Try to find a balance when evaluating yourself. It's easy to be deceived about areas in our own lives. "Oh, I'm not really that way!"—denial. Or, "I'm that way because . . ."—rationalization. Remember the story of the emperor's new clothes? The deluded ruler imagined that he was wearing luxurious, royal robes when he was really buck naked! And then—"out of the mouths of babes!"—a little boy blurted to the whole town that their great leader was ruling in the raw, and the emperor finally realized his reality. Self-deception had caused the king to deny the truth about himself.

We walk a fine line when it comes to accepting ourselves. On one hand, we want to have the peace of mind that comes with approving the way God made us. Some things we cannot change, and many things we won't want to. If you like yourself and feel satisfied, be thankful. On the other hand, some of us use self-acceptance as a crutch, saying, "That's just the way I am." We don't plan to change—it takes too much effort or a release of some pride to do so. Often, it doesn't matter how many people we hurt with that particular weakness. So be honest with yourself when you are evaluating what you would like to change and improve.

But be merciful too. More than likely, you have had times like the rest of us when you blow small imperfections out of proportion. You feel distraught over microscopic details about yourself or your life that, in your eyes, have grown into mountainous problems. If you mentioned these secrets to a friend, she'd only laugh that she hadn't noticed them!

The following poem would fit nicely into the Dreams and Goals section of our makeover notebooks. Written by Reinhold Niebuhr, the piece offers a balance between acceptance and change.

The Serenity Prayer

God, grant me the serenity
to accept the things I cannot change,
courage to change the things I can,
and wisdom to know the difference.

Worth a Thousand Words

We encourage you to take a photograph of yourself in the next few days—a full-length picture wearing one of your favorite outfits and hairstyles. This will serve as your "before" photo. You can date this, placing the picture in your "New You" Notebook. Photographs can help us notice our physical blind spots. Years ago, one of my (Cynthia's) friends looked at a photo of me and thoughtlessly remarked, "I didn't realize you were so broad across the beam." Oh, thanks so much! Fortunately, I didn't allow the criticism to get me down. Instead, I used it constructively. That remark showed me what I could not see—my caboose!—and I immediately went on a diet and exercise program to shape up.

Leave a space next to this recent photo for your "after" shot. This snapshot will record your progress in creating a whole new you. You and your friends will be truly amazed!

We can't take photographs of our spirits, but we can use a mirror to see what we are really like—the spiritual mirror of James 1:22–25:

> But prove yourselves doers of the word, and not merely hearers who delude themselves. For if anyone is a hearer of the word and not a doer, he is like a man who looks at his natural face in a mirror; for once he has looked at himself and gone away, he has immediately forgotten what kind of person he was. But one who looks intently at the perfect law, the law of liberty, and abides by it, not having become a forgetful hearer but an effectual doer, this man shall be blessed in what he does.

God's Word is the perfect hand tool to reflect our present shortcomings, our spiritual blind spots, those areas in our lives that are not pleasing to God. But with his help, we can change these blemishes on our character and bring them

Charity Chats

Okay, now it's my turn to speak. I've found that getting honest about the "real me" is one of the hardest yet most significant parts of the whole process. And it's that first plunging step into the murky depths of your secret soul that is often most intimidating. Sometimes it's easier if someone goes before you to "test the waters" first, and since my "secret soul" has already been ratted on (Thanks a lot, Mom!), I will be glad to jump into the deep end with you.

The following is an actual entry from my "New You" Notebook, written several years ago at the very beginning of my modeling pursuit, a time when I had to get painfully honest about the imbalance of my beauty:

> Lord, I know that the area of my life that is most disappointing to you is my self-esteem and my preoccupation with the physical.
>
> I am very hard on myself and hold up impossible standards of perfection that I am constantly falling short of.
>
> I am continually discouraged and disappointed.
>
> I am very insecure about my looks and only feel acceptable after I have devoted much time and effort into improving myself.
>
> I cannot accept myself as I am; my only confidence comes in bottles and brushes, tubes and techniques.
>
> Lord, I need your help! I need healing. I need your transformation!

These life-changing times of self-realization and spiritual transformation are what our journey toward the beautiful balance is all about. I dove in headfirst! Now it's your turn. Time to make a splash! Let's see what you're all about . . .

under the transforming grace of the Holy Spirit, becoming more and more like him.

Second Corinthians 3:18 says, "But we all, with unveiled face, beholding as in a mirror the glory of the Lord, are being

Cynthia Shares

In my notebook, I created a page titled "Ways I'm Not Like God/Jesus Christ." Below the title, I made two columns. Under the column "God/ Christ," I listed the attributes of the Lord that are recorded in his Word and that I've experienced personally. Under the column labeled "Me," I listed the characteristics of my life that don't measure up to God's glory—the traits I want to change. I bring these sinful areas before the Lord on a regular basis, in repentance. Also, I work at correcting them. I've been pleased to see some of these weaknesses changing in my life. My goal is to someday be like Christ. If this is also your ideal, you might like to include a similar page in your notebook. God has made each one of us so special. He has dreams for us too, and he will help us realize them when we respond to him.

transformed into the same image from glory to glory, just as from the Lord, the Spirit."

God's Word is like one of those fancy two-way mirrors: It reflects our imperfections on one side and the beauty and glory of our Lord and Savior, Jesus Christ, on the other. When we use this mirror every day, we are guaranteed to grow into the radiant beauties God has in mind.

Now let's move on to the other sections in our "New You" Notebooks.

Hair

Cut and paste magazine photos of hairstyles that might look good on you. You can pull these out and take them with you to the hairdresser's when you need a trim. In this section, you can also record the dates of your last permanent or color job. Keep track of products you have tried and the results. After reading our chapter on hair, create a schedule to implement a hair program specific to your needs.

Charity Chats

From experience, I can assure you that models don't have perfect skin. We get blemishes at all the wrong times just like everybody else. Makeup artists, however, have made concealing them a science. (And when that doesn't work, the photographers airbrush them out!) We use theatrical concealers, which you can purchase at a beauty supply store, and dab them on our blemishes. Since this is the chapter for makeover miracles, I'll share with you some things you can do to instantly transform yourself.

Cursed with a bad complexion? It can take several weeks or even months for a good skin program and nutrition plan to work. In the meantime, become the "queen of cover." Invest in a good foundation that matches your own skin exactly. Test a stripe on your jawline. If you can't tell where the foundation ends and your real skin begins, it's perfect! Foundations come in different blends: creams with an oil-base for dry skin; oil-free, water-based for oily skin; and a regular, oil-based formulation (often with sunscreen) for normal complexions. Foundation is a protection for your skin.

Foundation should glide on, using upward strokes. But go lightly. Cakey foundation "masks" are a major beauty-buster, in my opinion. To avoid foundation overkill, you can use a damp sponge for sheer but complete coverage. Blend at the jawline and be sure to include your neck. Allow foundation to dry, then brush your face in a downward motion with a light powder (matching your skin tone) to set foundation and remove any shine.

Skin

Record the problems you've experienced with your skin. Do you have frequent breakouts, continual shine, dry lines? Help is on the way! After reading chapter 4, you can design a skin-care regimen just for you. A glowing complexion will soon be yours with consistent care. Include your skin-care routine and the products that are working for you in this section. You can even paste in some "before" and "after" photos from the neck up, if you like. Take these in natural light with a bare face to reveal the true condition of your skin. You'll be pleasantly surprised after several weeks on the program.

Cosmetics

In this section, you can keep track of the glamour products you use. "Before" and "after" photos are fun here too. The first should be taken with a "naked" face; the second after you have your complete makeup on. Cynthia does this for clients, and they are thrilled when they see the difference. It's a good way to observe whether you like a certain makeup style or not. You can also cut and paste magazine photos that display a glamour look you want to try. Perhaps a model has eyes like yours. Try her techniques and see if you like the look on yourself. A special occasion may be in your near future. (Maybe that anniversary cruise!) Keeping a picture in your notebook will help you remember how you want to look for that event. As you read the chapters on making up eyes and lips (and their spiritual counterparts), you'll have enough ideas for your own book!

Figure

If you are like us, this will be the section of your notebook where you will spend lots of time. You can do many helpful things to enhance your ability to lose weight, tone up, and get fit. In our book *The Healthy Balance,* we share ways for you to evaluate your goals and devise your own diet and exercise plan. Whichever fitness program you choose, record it all in your notebook.

I (Cynthia) like to chart my weight loss with a graph and watch my weight go down, down, down. It's cheap entertain-

Charity Chats

For an instant lift, I like to add some color. You might want to try it too. Smile at yourself in the mirror. (You can do it!) Brush blusher on the "apples" of your cheeks, just under the irises of your eyes. Then sweep up across your cheekbones, and blend, blend, blend into your temples. Use a blush that matches your skin tone: if you have a yellow cast to your skin (like mine), choose a peachy blush. Women with a blue cast to their complexions (my mom, for example) look best with true pink or rose, depending on the depth of their coloring.

If I am scheduled for a photo shoot and I'm feeling heavier than usual, I contour under my cheekbones (suck your cheeks in) and jawline with a brownish-toned blush. It's very slimming, and you can even shape other features with it, like noses and cleavage. Less is always more with this technique, and be sure to blend.

ment! Every day that I exercise, I record what I did and how long I did it and if I stuck by my diet. I also record my weight every morning. Though I'm not obsessed with my weight, this practice seems to help me stay on track. When I'm seriously dieting, I also list what I eat each day, which really keeps me focused.

In this section of your notebook, you can compile all the foods that are on your "yes" list and those to avoid. You can also place a folder in your three-ring binder and add low-calorie recipes when you find them in magazines. Your meal plans can be included here too.

I (Charity) like to keep a journal of my food intake and exercise output, almost like a checkbook register. Sometimes I even comment on how I feel after exercise. "Did I feel weak, or did I want to run another two miles?" I gauge my progress this way.

"Before" and "after" photos will also demonstrate your improvement in this area. Glue in the "before" snapshot, leaving room next to it for your victory photograph. Take them in outfits that reveal your figure. If you are motivated visually, clip some photos of models in swimsuits—those can be inspirational too. Tape up an extra magazine photo on the fridge if that will help you stay away from between-meal snacks.

Before starting your fitness program, jot down your measurements: bust, hips, waist, upper arms, and upper thighs. You'll want to periodically record your improvements.

Models must work hard to keep their fit figures. We have friends who spend hours a day in the gym. Our bodies can take weeks and months to whip into shape. For instant improvement, however, stand up straight. So many of us walk into a room with our insecurities showing. Our heads are hanging down, our shoulders roll forward, bust lines sag, stomachs pooch out in one direction and fannies in another. This lack of confidence does terrible things for our figures. If you want an instantly improved body image, straighten up. Imagine that you have a string running through your head, through your body, down into your toes, and someone is pulling up on it. Or pretend you are being measured against the wall and you want to be taller. Best of all, as we said in chapter 1, remember that you are the daughter of the King of Kings. This will help you hold your head high. Imagine you are already wearing your crown and don't want it to slip!

Fashion

This section will end up packed with ideas as you establish your own unique style. If you aren't particularly adept at putting together complete outfits, snip pictures from magazines of models sporting the latest fashions—the ones that appeal to you and are appropriately modest, that is. You can even

Charity Chats

Personally, visual motivation really works for me. Here's how I used it to my advantage. I recently got married. It was very important to me to look and feel my best on my special day (and the seven extra-special days in Cancun that were to follow!). I cut out a picture of my favorite Victoria's Secret model in her underwear (the girl with the "ideal honeymoon body"), and I pasted her to the outside of my underwear drawer. That way, every day as I stood naked in front of the mirror, picking out my underwear, I had a visual reminder of my goal and could assess my progress.

Now remember, ladies, this method worked for me, a single gal, because I did not yet have a husband around to gawk at my sexy "paper doll." For those of you with this slight disadvantage, I strongly advise pasting the visual aid *inside* your underwear drawer!

include pictures of purses, shoes, and jewelry that call your name. You'll recognize these the next time you go to the department store, or you can bring these pages from your notebook with you when you shop. Start a list of clothing items and accessories that you need to complete your wardrobe. In addition, chapter 9 will help you discover the colors that best bring out your individual beauty. Be sure to include those colors in your "New You" Notebook, and you can take this list with you when you go shopping too.

Hands and Feet

Chapter 7 will give you ideas for beautiful hands and feet. Your hands and feet serve you well throughout the day and week. You'll learn ways to treat them well and help them look and feel better. In addition, jot down things that you would like to accomplish with your hands, places that you'd like your feet to take you.

Cynthia Shares

I'm a living example of a makeover, a transformation of both body and soul. My mother loves to tell the story of my high school years. I considered myself an athlete. I was a runner and sort of a tomboy—I even picked out my wedding dress in track shoes! On Saturdays, I would hang around the house all scroungy: T-shirt, cutoffs, long hair twisted up in a barrette, no makeup. Then the phone would ring and a certain young man (my high school sweetheart and future husband) would call for a date. Up the stairs I would bound, two at a time. An hour later, I'd float down to my awaiting beau a different girl, and my mother would laugh. My hair was styled beautifully, my makeup perfectly applied, and I was dressed like a fashion model. As I matured (and after winning a couple of queen pageants and embarrassing myself when people didn't recognize me without makeup), I decided I'd try to look my best all of the time, and not just on special occasions.

While in college, I came to grips with some areas of my spirit that needed a makeover. Severe depression, fear, negativity, and low self-worth threatened to destroy me. But then I made Jesus Christ Lord of my life. He gently took me through a renewal plan that I'll explain as we go along. It was the best thing that ever happened to me! Like my mother says, I am a different girl. A girl who reflects the light, life, and love of her Savior.

Miscellaneous

As we said, this is your notebook, and you can include any sections you want. Add those that will be helpful in your individual life. An expense record and file for purchases; a date book with calendar; lists of books you want to read or have read; goals that you have for personal growth, such as community college classes or job enrichment courses. Your notebook will be as individual and creative as your life. In the past few months, Charity's notebook held a section for weddings (as she planned

Charity Chats

Clothing designers want to show off the newest line in their catalogs. It's their best work, but that doesn't always mean it's ideal for the model.

I remember having to model a hideous, white, plus-sized jogging suit for a sports designer. Not so good—I'm a petite model. Sport clothes usually look best with sport shoes; the only shoes I brought were high heels. Regardless, I had to fulfill my obligation.

So I slipped my head into the top . . . and it swallowed me alive! You can imagine my embarrassment as I tip-toed out of the changing tent for the shoot. I looked like the "Abominable Snowwoman"! Trust me, I did not feel good about myself while wearing it.

But think about outfits that make you feel so good that you can't help but smile when you're wearing them. Maybe it's the bright, cheerful color, the silky feel of the cloth, the glamorous style, or the perfect fit. Whatever it is, you wear it well, and it makes you look and feel beautiful. That's what is important. As you search for photos of outfits for your notebook (and clothes for your closet), remember this approach.

hers), and more recently, Cynthia added some pages for lessons in Spanish, a language she'd determined to master this year.

Soul Care

Your "New You" Notebook should have a section just for your spirit. This will be a sacred place for you to go each day. Have your Bible reading schedule or Bible study there. Also include prayer lists for yourself and your loved ones. Jot down names of those who need Christ. Have a spot to record and date God's incredible answers. Include in this section favorite Scriptures that have touched your heart, and why. You will want to record your experiences, thoughts, and feelings on your exciting journey. Have journal pages ready for this. Write out your testimony, and know what you believe.

Our salvation is the foundation for a beautiful spirit, and our continual loveliness in Christ is guaranteed. Philippians 1:6 promises: "For I am confident of this very thing, that He who began a good work in you will perfect it until the day of Christ Jesus."

Isn't it great to know that our spiritual makeovers will continue until we are perfect in God's sight? He will never give up on us. And he has so much more planned for our future than we can even imagine.

Don't be afraid of surrendering to an overhaul at the hands of the Creator, the Expert in spiritual beauty. He is the Potter, you are the clay. Allow him to have his way in your life, and you will never regret it. Like the ladies in our makeover classes, you will be more than thrilled at the results!

3

The Mane Thing

Having a bad hair day? Or maybe it's been a "bad hair year"! Would you like to get your confidence back? That's what this chapter will give you—something to smile about. Even right now, you may be saying that you hate your hair, that you can't do a thing with it. But you can learn to accept the hair God gave you and learn to make the most of it.

Most women feel this way about their hair—we always want what we don't have. It's either too curly or too straight, too dark or too light, and sooner or later, too gray. So in this chapter, we have come to a subject we can all agree on. Everyone wants beautiful hair. Women may opt out when it comes to makeup, preferring a natural look. They may choose not to spend time or money on manicures and pedicures. But we have yet to meet a woman who doesn't care about her hair.

And for good reason. Hair is a vital component of our femininity. When it's gone, we feel less womanly. Terri, a friend of ours who suffered with cancer, put off having her first surgery because she didn't want to lose her long, blonde hair. It was a part of the young woman's identity. Then, after two brain surgeries, chemotherapy, and radiation that left her hairless, Terri bought a very full, bleached blonde wig. We didn't recognize her the first time she wore it. Terri could have won a Dolly Parton look-alike contest! It made her feel better, though, and we understood. Terri's choices may seem foolish, but having worked with women for so many years, we know that her feelings and fears are universal. In some small way, our hair defines who we are.

Finding a Frame to Fit

We need to think of our hair as a frame for the artwork of our face. Think about the importance of a frame to a painting. Several years ago, after a Southern California book signing, the bookstore owner gave me (Cynthia) a lovely painting of a mother kneeling by her bed as she prayed for her children. The picture reminded me of my own commitment to raise godly children. My husband and I set out to find just the right frame to enhance it, but we finally designed a custom frame that suited the painting perfectly. In the same way that a frame adorns the beauty of an artist's masterpiece, your hair frames God's creative genius—your lovely face—accenting your own unique beauty.

Is anything more eye-catching than soft, healthy, shimmering hair? Since time began, luxurious hair has been a symbol of vitality and sensuality. How about you? Is your hair your "crowning glory"? Or are you disappointed with your lackluster locks? Maybe your hair is dry and brittle from too many perms and color jobs. Or the opposite problem might plague your scalp, which you think contains more oil than a Persian Gulf nation! Perhaps you don't like the color. Gray got you down? Have you had the same style since

1975—you know, the one that matches your high school yearbook photo? Feel like a change, but unsure what would suit you best?

If you answered yes to any of these questions, you might be wondering, "What can I do about it?" Lots! There is hope for helpless hair. No matter what the health of your hair now, it can improve. If you don't like the shape of things, a new style could be the way to go. Create a section in your "New You" Notebook labeled "Hair." Jot down the changes you'd like to see. Put it all in a time frame. Remember, goals undated are goals undone.

> "True beauty comes from within— but gorgeous hair can't hurt!"
>
> —television commercial for Conair Pro/Rusk hair products

Clip and paste into that section pictures of styles that you like and think would be flattering. Record tips and information that will help make the most of your tresses. And think positive. By practicing the information in the following pages, every day can be a great hair day!

Hair Typology 101

Discovering what type of hair you have begins your journey toward a marvelous mane. Answer these questions, and jot your evaluation in your workbook.

1. When I touch my hair, it feels almost like:
   a. strands of silk.
   b. an actual head of human hair.
   c. boar bristles.
2. The strands of my hair are:
   a. small in diameter.

    b. medium-sized.

    c. large in diameter.

3. My hair is:

    a. fragile, thin, and delicate, with hardly any body. It lies limply on my head.

    b. soft to the touch, full, with good body and manageability.

    c. Thick, with lots of weighty volume. It grows away from my scalp.

4. No matter what products I use, the day after shampooing, my hair:

    a. has less static and more shine and generally feels better than just after a wash.

    b. hasn't changed much since I shampooed the day before.

    c. is a grease pit, dark and dank. Must be washed again!

If you answered questions 1 through 3 with "a" answers, you have fine hair, and more than likely, it's thin. If you gave "c" answers, you probably have a thick, coarse head of hair; "b" answers indicate a tendency toward normalcy. Question 4 deals with your scalp's oil production or lack of it. "A" answers are telltale for dry hair; "c" answers are obviously oily; and "b" answers again indicate a normal, healthy head of hair. Fine or coarse, thin or thick, dry or oily—it's your hair, and you can win with it. Here are some rules to help you play the Manage Your Mane game.

The Rules of the Game

We have three cardinal rules for loving the hair God gave you:

1. Accept the type of hair you were given at birth and work with it. Extreme changes can be made—for instance, very straight hair can be curled with permanent waves, and curly hair can be straightened. The dark-haired beauty can be transformed into a Marilyn Monroe bombshell. But these kinds of alterations take time, effort, and money to keep up. Are you willing to pay the price? If not, there are ways to make the most of what you have, and we'll talk about them in this chapter.

2. To look good, hair must be taken care of. Hair is not a living thing. It's an appendage. Inside your scalp are little follicles where the hair strands are alive. As soon as they push out into the cruel world, they die and begin to deteriorate. Hair closest to the scalp is healthiest. Hair longer than a half inch can accumulate damage from sun, environment, illness, and abuse. Your job as a hair owner is to counteract that damage.

3. The cut is the most important factor in how your hair looks—and in how you feel about it. Think about how you feel when your hairstyle gets out of shape, straggly, and draggy. You feel draggy, right? But as soon as you get a trim, you perk right up, and so does your appearance.

In this chapter, we'll cover these three rules, working backwards.

A Cut Above

Need to know how to get the right cut? Find the right stylist! Here's how.

Search for a trustworthy stylist who is talented with her or his scissors. Every hairdresser has areas of expertise, so when you want a great cut, don't go to one who is famous for weaves. Get references from friends. Or if you see a stranger with a great cut, ask her name and the name of her stylist.

Cynthia Shares

When you find your stylist, make sure he or she has a knack for knowing what style looks good on you. You might take a picture into the shop, showing what hairdo you'd like. But will it look good for your face shape and with your texture of hair? When I worked in a shop, women would bring in magazine photos of their favorite actresses and say, "I want you to make me look like her." I'd joke back, "This is a hair cut, Suzy, not plastic surgery." The woman got the joke, laughed, and hopefully also got the point. Not every style is suited for every person. And the style might look like the star, but the face might not. Just be prepared in advance for some variations.

She will most likely be happy to give you the information—we girls love networking. Then it's easy to make an appointment with the woman's stylist and simply say, "I want a cut just like Sara's!"

It's preferable that your stylist has been working for years (maybe even the salon owner) but has kept up-to-date. Be sure your hairdresser is willing to listen to your desires and the explanation of your lifestyle. And remember, along with some degree of talent and skill, a good stylist has a generous heart. He or she will fix any problems free of charge.

Facing Up

You can find hairstyles that look good for every face shape. To determine the shape of your face, pull your hair back completely. No bangs please. Look into a mirror. Is your face round, oval, heart-shaped, square, rectangular, or diamond? If you have a hard time figuring out your face shape, take a bar of soap and draw around your reflection directly onto the mirror. Does that help?

Short, round faces benefit from a style with long, slimming lines. Thin, longer faces need widening with a hairstyle that has fullness at the sides. And consider the length of your neck. Women with short necks look better with shorter hair, or updos. Extra long, thin necks need hair to fill in. Also, consider prominent features. A large nose needs balance with fullness in the back of the head. A receding chin does too. Got gorgeous eyes? A fringe of bangs might play them up big-time.

Keep track of all these self-discoveries in your notebook. Here's a fun assignment: Go to a grocery or drugstore, and glance through the latest hairstyle magazines. When you find a book with lots of styles that you like, buy it. Remember to consider your face shape. Did you find a style (or styles) in the magazine that you simply must try? Cut out the picture and paste it into your notebook. You can take it to your stylist and ask for that particular cut. You've done the preliminary work and have more of a chance at being completely thrilled when you walk out the salon door.

Are you particularly adept at styling your own hair? If not, have it professionally done just after a new cut. It's worth the extra money. You can watch your hairdresser's maneuvers and duplicate them at home. Be sure to ask any questions that you have. A good hairdresser will always supply you with the information you need to look your best.

Styling with the Best of Them

Your perfect style is determined by more than the shape of your face. The type of hair that you have plays a huge part. Is your fine hair oily and thin? Thick, coarse, and dry at the ends?

Straight or curly? Has your normal hair been damaged by too much processing? We'll cover these topics one by one.

Oily Hair

Remember, hair itself doesn't produce oil—the scalp does. This is where you need to attack the problem. The oil seeps down the hair shaft. Not long after a shampoo, your hair is once again heavy, greasy, and even matted, right? Extreme oiliness is a problem for anyone. But a woman with fine, thin hair needs special help.

We recommend a short, simple style that can be washed every day. Hair can be shampooed as often as necessary in warm water (hot stimulates your oil glands to produce more oil), so don't worry about the frequency. However, do use a gentle shampoo that has good sudsing action. Industrial-strength cleansers are not necessary, in spite of the grease. And don't use one of the all-in-one products—shampoo and conditioner in one bottle. They cause buildup on your hair.

Shampoo twice. The first time will remove the dirt, oil, and any products left on your hair. The second shampoo adds volume. If your hair is short, one shampoo will do and you may not need a conditioner at all. You are continually cutting off the damaged ends, and your hair is short enough to keep conditioned with natural oil. Longer hair will probably need an oil-free detangler before combing out. Apply it only to the ends and length of the hair. Avoid getting conditioner on your scalp.

Oiliness is caused by hormones, those little biological chemicals that are a mixed blessing. You won't be able to stop the oil production. But with this plan, you will be able to control its effect on your hair.

Dry Hair

Your scalp can be naturally dry, or you may be experiencing weather-induced dryness. In either case, shampoo twice a week to rid your hair and scalp of accumulated hair products. Use comfortable warm water (hot can dry the ends). Then condition with a rich conditioner made for frequent use. Avoid products that are oil-based—these cling to the scalp and hair. If your hair is fine, this is bad news! Massage the conditioner into the ends of your hair, and then up into the scalp. Leave on one minute. Rinse thoroughly. To moisturize a dry, itchy scalp, rub some oil or facial moisturizer into your scalp before bed. Generously shampoo your scalp the following morning. Rinse well and enjoy a reprieve from a flaky, dry head.

Damaged Hair

Damaged hair is usually dry. The ends are split, and often the hair is damaged all the way up its shaft. It feels like straw and appears lifeless with little or no shine. These truly are "dread-locks"! You can regain normal hair in two steps: first, undo the damage, and second, prevent it from happening again.

The quickest, easiest way to get healthy hair again is to cut off all the damage. This is extreme. But from experience, we know it works. We've had horrid perms, and the only solution has been to cut off the permed hair and start fresh. We can't stand it when our hair starts feeling damaged on the ends, can you? Fortunately, hair grows back rather quickly, at a rate of one-half inch a month.

After you've cut, you need to prevent. Two of the best preventions are deep conditioning and detangling.

Deep Conditioning

The next best thing to a cut is to deep condition once a week with a restructuring conditioner (ask your hairdresser or at a beauty supply store). This is left on the hair for ten or twenty minutes at a time. Adding heat to this regimen increases its effectiveness by opening up the cuticle of the hair so the conditioner can penetrate.

Shampoo as suggested for dry hair. Always towel-dry without wringing or stretching your hair. Wet hair is very vulnerable, especially if it's fine or damaged. Squeeze a good dollop of conditioner (about a tablespoon) into your hands, rub them together, then spread throughout your hair, beginning at the damaged ends. Place a plastic shower cap or baggie over your hair and sit under a very warm dryer for ten to twenty minutes. Or you can wrap your head with a warm, moist, steamy towel. After the conditioning treatment, rinse thoroughly.

A deep conditioner doesn't have to be expensive. For hair treatments, we don't have to look any farther than our kitchens. The Bible commands us not to be drunk with wine, but it says nothing about using alcohol as a hair product! Flat beer works very well poured through your freshly washed and towel-dried hair, becoming a great conditioner and setting lotion. (Don't worry—you won't smell like you've just come from a bar. The odor of the alcohol fades fast.)

To lighten your hair a little, lemon and vodka will do the trick. Blonde models often sit in the sun sporting this little mixture. But take it from experience, condition well after this treatment. The acid content in lemon juice can dry out your hair in no time. Want to be a "champagne" blonde? Pour some of the bubbly through your locks for light, lovely highlights.

If you're a brunette, brew some strong coffee, cool it, then pour it through your hair. Leave it on for thirty minutes. Rinse out and style as usual. Notice new glistening highlights!

Chamomile tea, cooled and worn for twenty minutes, then rinsed out, adds brightness to dark blonde and light brown heads.

Old seltzer water, and of course the ever-popular vinegar, will strip hair of product buildup. Mix with water and use (occasionally) before final rinse.

For conditioning, all of us can use mashed banana or avocado. Massage into damp hair. Allow it to condition for fifteen minutes, then rinse. The natural oils in these fruits are the conditioning agents. Mayonnaise applied in the same way also works very well. The oil conditions and the protein-rich eggs add shine. But do wash out thoroughly.

If your hair is dry at the ends or your scalp is feeling dry and itchy, try a homemade hot-oil treatment: Heat a little olive oil or almond oil in a pan. Massage into damp hair and scalp. Allow to penetrate for twenty minutes, then shampoo and rinse.

God has a pantry full of goodies that will make us pretty. Try some of these suggestions and see if they work for you. Don't forget to put God's bounty on the inside too. Beautiful hair grows out of your own good healthy eating habits.

Detangling

Prevention of hair damage begins with the very next procedure: your after-shampoo comb-out. We cringe when watching some women comb out their wet, fragile hair. Do *not* use a brush to detangle. It will break hair all the way up the hair shaft. However, on dry hair, the opposite is true—don't use a comb. You can hear the crackling of breaking hair as women rip through their long, dry locks with a comb. When your hair is dry, use a soft brush instead. Never start at the top and work down. This will break the hair too. With a wide-toothed comb or a hair pick, begin to detangle at the ends of your damp hair, working your way to the top.

Blow-drying and Styling

To provide volume and lift to your hair, try bending over from the waist and blow-dry with your head hanging upside down. Your hair will get more volume by blow-drying it against the direction that it grows. Use your fingers to comb through and lift as you blow. To prevent damage, hold the blow-dryer six inches from your hair. When your hair is nearly dry, you can begin to style it, using a brush (regular or round) to shape. With your dominant hand, pull the brush through the hair while the other hand blows the air in the direction you want the hair to go. For volume, lift and curl. Hair needs to be slightly damp to get the desired shape. Use some mousse or gel, if needed. These will also tame any flyaway hairs.

Finish up your style with some strategically placed hot rollers or use a curling iron. The fatter the iron, the bigger and looser the curl. Some rollers and rods only add body. Make sure the ends are smooth when you curl the hair strand around the utensil. Then roll her up! If your hair is damaged, use these appliances sparingly.

If you were born with naturally stick-straight hair, you're probably a big fan of curling irons and hot rollers. Try the following methods to combat the damage that these tools do:

- Do regular hot-oil treatments.
- Use hot rollers for special-occasion "do's" until hair damage is reversed.
- Switch from "heavy metal" rollers to the newer, velvet-covered type.

When you remove the rollers, turn your head upside down once more and give a quick, gentle brush-through to loosen curl and add volume. Then you can use a brush or pick to style your hair. If you choose, a final spritz with hairspray will keep your "do" done for hours.

Matriarchal Myths

You've gotta love Grandma, but definitely forget some of the old wives' tales she's told you:

1. *"Brush a hundred strokes a night for healthy, shiny hair."* Think again, Grams. Handling your hair in any shape or form damages the cuticle. Always work on your hair gently, only as often as necessary, and then with soft brushes and wide-tooth combs that won't tear.
2. *"You look so cute in a ponytail, dear, and it's the best way to keep that hair off your face."* Not! Ponytails can be damaging. Ladies and girls pull them tightly away from their faces, causing permanent loss at their hairline. In addition, they use bands that break the hair where it's gathered in the back. Never use a regular rubber band, like the ones that wrap around the daily newspaper! If you must wear a ponytail (as we often do when we're working around the house), pull the hair away from the face loosely. Tie your tail with a stretchy, coated band, a scrunchy, or a soft ribbon.
3. *"Sweetie, the only reason you are having those problems (e.g., dandruff, lice, etc.) is because you aren't clean enough."* Whatever! Unfortunately, the cleanest people on earth can have a problem with these pesti-

lences. Dandruff has several causes. It's now believed that true dandruff may be caused by a yeast organism that normally lives on the scalp. An imbalance develops, the cause unknown at this time, and the yeast overgrows on the scalp, resulting in the detestable flakiness. Our recommendation is to use a shampoo containing ketoconazole, either over-the-counter or prescription. Ketoconazole is an antifungal drug that will get to the root of your problem.

Some flakes are not dandruff but simply buildup of products on the hair. We all experience this on occasion. If you do too, use a clarifying shampoo about once a week to rid your hair of accumulated gunk.

Lice, in the same way, are no respecter of persons. Rich, poor, clean or not, you acquire a headful of these tiny pests by close encounters with someone who is infested. Prevention is best. Avoid using others' combs, brushes, and other hair care utensils. Don't share pillows or hats either. It's nice to be close, but touching heads with someone who has lice is a risky practice. Train your kids on these matters—the head you save may be your own.

If you get the bug, however, see a doctor immediately for a prescription of lindane, which will kill the lice on contact. From experience, playing around with homemade and over-the-counter remedies just gives the critters more time to multiply. The lindane must be reapplied several days later to rid your hair of any hatched eggs. Do not overuse, however, as the medication is quite potent. Follow your doctor's directions carefully. Between applications, you have your work cut out for you. Launder all bed linens, including blankets and comforters, in hot water, then dry in a hot dryer. Do the same to any clothes that came in contact with the carrier. If something can't be laundered, it can be sealed in a plastic bag for a week to kill any bugs. Vacuum the whole house thoroughly, especially carpets and fabric-covered sofas and chairs.

4. *"I don't know why you are losing your hair, child. No one else in the family has ever had that problem. Why, when I was in my fifties, I still had a full head of hair."* Remember, Grandma's memory may not be as sharp as it once was. She forgets that Uncle Joe has been bald as a billiard ball since his early thirties. The most common cause of hair loss is genetic. Termed *androgenetic alopecia* (hereditary hair loss), this problem affects 40 percent of women. Unfortunately, female hair loss usually begins as it does for men—at the hairline, working its way back across the crown. The cause is genetically programmed hormones (androgens) that, little by little, erode the hair follicles, resulting in finer, thinner hair until finally . . . it's gone. Fortunately it's rare for a woman to lose all of her hair like a man. Some hair loss is related to pregnancy and other hormone-related changes. These problems usually cease when hormones regulate. Stress can cause hair loss, too. Called *alopecia areata*, this can happen because stress of any kind can trigger the immune system to begin attacking hair follicles.

Some of the Israelite women had the problem of hair today, gone tomorrow. According to Isaiah 3:16–17, something worse than bad genes caused their hair to fall out:

Moreover, the LORD said, "Because the daughters of Zion are proud,
And walk with heads held high and seductive eyes,
And go along with mincing steps

And tinkle the bangles on their feet,
Therefore the Lord will afflict the scalps of the daughters of
Zion with scabs,
And the LORD will make their foreheads bare."

Stay humble, girls. And step along briskly. No seductive, mincing strolls. We want to keep a full head of hair!

Today we have several other hair loss remedies in addition to humility (an always desirable trait). Minoxidil products (available at drugstores) have been proven to grow hair in 40 to 63 percent of women who religiously use it. Applied topically, the lotion is messy and can cause some facial hair growth. But most women agree they'd rather tackle the problem of hair on their face than none on their heads. Also, if you want to keep the regrowth, you must keep applying the Minoxidil for life.

Color Me Beautiful

Have you ever wondered if blondes really do have more fun? As a lifelong and very committed natural brunette, I (Cynthia) wouldn't know. But golden girl Charity seems to attract a lot of attention! Maybe you'd like to discover for yourself if blondes live more exciting lives. Whether it's best to go lighter or change your hair color at all depends on your complexion.

Surely you've seen a dark-skinned, dark-eyed beauty with colorless bleached hair. It just doesn't fit, does it? She looks lifeless and washed out, often having to compensate with more makeup. It seems the Father knew best which color would perfectly suit his lovely daughter.

On the other hand, some women began life as sunshiny towheads, only to grow darker and duller over the years. Let's blame this condition (and all our other weaknesses and flaws, right?) on the fall and do something about it. Lightening hair can be a fresh, uplifting change. This one alteration adds a lift to your appearance (and spirits), giving you a coveted glow.

The authors recommend having your hair bleached professionally. To echo the sentiments of Truvy (played by Dolly Parton), hair salon owner in the film *Steel Magnolias:* "I never trust a woman who does her own hair!" All kidding aside, stripping color from hair to precisely the right shade is a science. Finding the correct shade of toner is an art. You've probably seen as many brassy home jobs walking around town as we have. Hire a trained "artist" to bleach your hair. Afterward, remember to deep condition and trim damaged ends regularly. And please, keep your roots done!

If you're looking for something a little less dramatic (and damaging) with less upkeep, try a frost or weave. You can ask for a full or partial weave or frost. And your hairdresser will find just the right shade of toner to suit your complexion. Frosts and weaves last longer between appointments so they save you money too.

For those of us with darker tresses, adding highlights will perk up our coloring. Red or auburn streaks look good on women with golden tones to their skin and eyes. If you're like Cynthia, with ivory skin (or a blue cast to your complexion) and light eyes, ash-tones are best.

Got Gray?

There is nothing more striking than dazzling white hair or a silvery-gray head. The Bible even says that the honor of old men (and women) is their gray hair (Proverbs 20:29). Scripture talks about white hair symbolizing the wisdom that we have gained from years of living. Most of us, however, are covering up our wisdom! In our society, unlike cultures in other parts of the world, we don't value the old and wise. The younger women don't seek out the older, wiser, more experienced women. Instead, the older women are trying to be like the young girls. This is backwards, and not the way God planned it. We Christian women need to take a stand and be proud of the years God has given us.

But if you would like to be proud of your years without being so flamboyant about them (i.e., flaunting a gray crown), or if you need a little less honor and a little more pizzazz, you can cover the gray yourself with any of the simple kits available at drugstores. Here are a few tips to see you through the procedure:

1. Gather all the supplies suggested on the box into your work area. Include some Vaseline or gel to spread along hairline and nape of neck to avoid staining.
2. Do a strand test to be sure of color and your skin's reaction.
3. Follow directions to the letter.
4. Color roots first, leave on the recommended amount of time, then pull through to ends of hair for the last ten minutes or so. (The porous hair absorbs more color faster.) During touch-ups, you can do a soap-cap on the ends, just like they do in a salon: After roots are processed, mix the remaining color with some shampoo. Shampoo your whole head with this, leaving on for five to ten minutes. Then rinse, shampoo, and rinse again.
5. Wear old, dark clothes, use old towels, and while processing, sit and read a book, do your nails, or watch the news. We have ruined more things (even a carpet) trying to do our hair while also doing housework.

6. Record the date that you colored your hair in your date book. Include the results. You'll need to redo each month or so, and you'll learn things about your own hair that you'll want to remember for next time.

Curl Up and Cry

How many of you have felt like crying after you've invested in a permanent? Both of us have! Sometimes it's too curly, even frizzy. And once the fuzz is there—like the name says—it's permanent. The only way to get rid of it is to cut it off. Or the opposite is true—it has little curl and you're thinking, *I paid that for this?* You're actually worse off now because not only is your hair stick-straight but it's damaged too.

In a word, we want to warn you about home perms: Don't! You're playing with harsh chemicals, and you can end up with a heartbreaking mess. You know the disclaimer that flashes during television magic shows, "Don't try this at home." We feel the same way about straightening, which is probably the most damaging of procedures that you can do to your hair.

So this is our recommendation about perms and chemical processing: If you must perm or straighten, get it done professionally. Notice perms around you, and ask who the stylist was. At your appointment, suggest a soft wave. When I (Cynthia) worked as a hairdresser, I often permed first, then cut the style afterwards. (If the hair was long going short, I would cut to shoulders or chin first, perm, then cut in the layers afterwards.) This trimmed off any fuzzy, damaged ends and created a soft, natural-looking wave.

Thankfully, the 1990s and beyond have brought us wash-and-wear hair. We have some wonderful styles today that don't need much care or curl and that work with the type of hair you have. All you have to do is shampoo and blow-dry.

Heavenly Hair

I (Cynthia) was born with thick, easy-to-manage hair but really hadn't given it much thought until I began to lose it. We humans always appreciate something more after it's gone, don't we? Of course, we'll do everything we can to preserve our assets, including our hair. But we also have to trust God with all that concerns us. After all, he knows and cares for us so much that he has every hair on our heads numbered. Can't you just hear his heavenly management team looking down with record book in hand, "Uh oh, there goes hair number 3,465, falling fast. Looks like hair number 3,582 will fill that follicle now." What a job God has in loving us!

In Matthew 10:28–31 and again in Luke 12:6–7, Jesus reassures us that our heavenly Father considers us very valuable. Using the example that God even has every hair on our head numbered, Jesus demonstrates some key attributes of his Father. God is the Creator. He is omniscient (all-knowing), omnipotent (all-powerful), and omnipresent (always with us). Considering the fact that we lose a hundred hairs a day and are continually growing new hairs, keeping track of all that fuzz on every human past, present, and future is a task for a mighty big God.

Psalm 139 expresses these truths so eloquently:

O LORD, you have searched me and you know me.
You know when I sit and when I rise;
     you perceive my thoughts from afar.
You discern my going out and my lying down,
     you are familiar with all my ways.

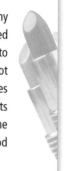

Charity Chats

I decided to stop worrying so much about glamour and start loving my hair as it is naturally. I finally grew my hair out and got one of those layered un-styles, à la Gwyneth Paltrow or Faith Hill. It gave my hair a chance to renew itself after years of blow-dryers and hot rollers. Now my hair is not nearly as big as it used to be, but it is so much healthier, and that makes me feel like a "natural beauty." If you have curly hair, get a cut that accents the body and wave. If it's straight, opt for a style that shows off its shine and silkiness. This is an example of when it is wise to accept what God gave you and go with it!

Before a word is on my tongue
    you know it completely, O Lord.
You hem me in—behind and before;
    you have laid your hand upon me.
Such knowledge is too wonderful for me,
    too lofty for me to attain.
Where can I go from your Spirit?
    Where can I flee from your presence?
If I go up to the heavens, you are there;
    if I make my bed in the depths, you are there.
If I rise on the wings of the dawn,
    if I settle on the far side of the sea,
even there your hand will guide me,
    your right hand will hold me fast. . . .
For you created my inmost being;
    you knit me together in my mother's womb.
I praise you because I am fearfully and wonderfully made;
    your works are wonderful,
    I know that full well.
My frame was not hidden from you
    when I was made in the secret place.
When I was woven together in the depths of the earth,

your eyes saw my unformed body.
All the days ordained for me
were written in your book
before one of them came to be.

verses 1–10, 13–16 NIV

Think about this. God knows you and me intimately. He watches our every move and knows what we are going to say even before the words come out of our mouths. In our case, we're sure he often thinks, "Oh no, there Cynthia goes . . . about to put her foot in her mouth." Or, "It's hard to believe Charity is going to say that . . . again!"

God is even aware of our thoughts. I (Cynthia) sometimes tell the Lord, "Oh well, Lord, I may as well tell you. You know what I'm thinking anyway." There is nowhere that we can go in the earth—on, above, or below—to get away from God's presence. He is always with us. If we are obeying him, this should be a comforting thought.

In his power, God planned and created us while we were still a gleam in our father's eye, continuing his work while we were in our mother's wombs. At birth, we were exactly as he had planned us way back at the beginning of time. Our family used to sing a song: "I was in his mind before the worlds were formed . . . I was in his mind . . . because he loves me." The Creator was thinking of each of us, individually, imagining you and me just as he designed us before the foundation of the earth.

God is love. It's his nature. And his love is unconditional. God's commitment to us is not dependent on anything we do. It's not just a warm, fuzzy feeling either. God's love is a powerful force, an active love, best demonstrated by the fact that he sent his Son, Jesus, to die for us while we were undeserving sinners (see Rom. 5:8). What greater proof of God's unconditional, committed love can there be than that?

The Father thought each of us was so valuable that he paid a high price to buy us back from the Enemy. He gave us full rights as his children, adopting us into his family. First John 3:1 says, "See how great a love the Father has bestowed on us, that we would be called children of God; and such we are." I am his child, the daughter of the King of Kings! And so are you, if you have received Jesus Christ as your own Savior and Lord.

Just as surely as you are your father's daughter and I am my father's, we who have received Jesus Christ are the beloved children of God. Romans 8:15–16 says that the Holy Spirit reassures us that we truly are children of God and that we have such an intimate relationship with our heavenly Father that we can even call him "Abba" or "Daddy." ("Abba" is the affectionate name Hebrew children call their daddies.)

God loves you like a perfect Father. He's proud of you, his creation, just as you are proud of your own children and love them more than life itself. Don't you want to give your kids wonderful things? Our heavenly Father wants to give you, his precious daughter, good gifts (Matt. 7:11). He even plans some of your heart's desires (Ps. 37:4)—and we have noticed that he will often change our hearts to desire what he wants to give. A winning plan! He wants only the best for you, and he's willing to sacrifice to provide it. Meditate on this for a while, and praise God for it!

The Main Thing

As beautiful women, we want to find the balance for our lives. To do so, we must prioritize, focusing on the important things. We need to know our one purpose in life. How do we decide what that one most important thing is?

In the movie *City Slickers,* Billy Crystal's character is on a midlife journey to find the meaning of life. He becomes friends with a cowboy named Curly. To Billy, this crusty old cowpoke embodies all the wisdom of the ages. Billy asks him what is the most important thing in life. A man of few words, Curly holds up one finger and growls, "This one thing . . ." That's his whole answer: "This one thing . . ." Curly dies soon after that. Billy has to find out for himself what "this one thing" is.

For the Christian, the main thing is to always remember that God loves us and sent his Son Jesus Christ to die for us so that we might have an eternal relationship with him. Jesus came willingly because he loved us so much. There's a lot of love going back and forth in this relationship. Mary, the sister of Martha, experienced this love. She sat at the feet of Jesus, listening to him, enjoying and adoring her Lord. Martha complained that Mary should be serving him instead. But Jesus stopped her. "Martha, Martha, you are worried and bothered about so many things," he soothed. "But only one thing is necessary, for Mary has chosen the good part, and it shall not be taken away from her" (Luke 10:38–42).

As believers, our purpose in life is to love God and enjoy him forever. When we focus on "this one thing," on loving Jesus Christ, cherishing him almost as much as he cherishes us, we'll be beautifully balanced women of God.

4

More Than Skin Deep

Would you like to have softer, smoother, younger-looking skin?

We all start out with a beautiful complexion—skin as soft as the proverbial baby's bottom, our mothers have assured us. But time, neglect, and the environment take their toll, leaving us with varying degrees of lined, rough, sun-damaged skin. We have good news for you though. No matter how your skin looks and feels today, with a little TLC it can look and feel a whole lot better! We have seen faces ravaged by the sun turn radiant and glowing from the benefits of a good skin care program. What you do for your skin today will make a dramatic difference in the way you look tomorrow. In this chapter, we share beauty secrets that will improve your complexion no matter what your age. But first, let's go over a few important details about your skin.

Your skin, fearfully and wonderfully made, has three layers. The epidermis is the outer layer of the skin, the one that the outside world sees. It's amazing to think that this exterior layer is only 1/1,000 of an inch thick, yet your appearance depends on its condition. The epidermis is a protective covering, screening out harmful environmental onslaughts that come against your face and body. New cells are constantly formed in this layer, but as we age, cell reproduction slows down.

The second layer is the dermis. This is the skin's major support system containing blood vessels, sebaceous (oil) glands, and hair follicles, all deeply rooted in the dermis. This layer also produces collagen, a protein that keeps your skin resilient and youthful, and elastin, another protein component that creates elasticity, causing the skin to snap back in shape when stretched. These are the two main elements that are affected by sun and gravity.

The subdermis is the innermost layer of the skin. This is where the fatty tissue and muscle of your face reside.

The treatments that we'll share in this chapter will condition your skin's epidermis, or outer later. It will be helpful to first diagnose what type of skin you have. You can record your findings in your "New You" Notebook, along with the skin-care program perfect for your skin type.

Skin Type Pop Quiz

1. Look into a mirror and smile. Do you see
   a. laugh lines around your eyes, mouth, or cheeks that aren't funny?
   b. visible pores but a basically smooth texture?
   c. shine so bright you need to wear shades?
2. Touch your face. Does your skin feel
   a. tight and taut and possibly flaky?
   b. smooth and soft, neither oily or dry?
   c. bumpy with blemishes and blackheads and oily to the touch?

3. Five hours after cleansing, will your skin become
   a. very dry to moderately dry?
   b. basically unchanged and moist?
   c. very oily?
4. Blemishes, along with blackheads and whiteheads,
   develop on your skin
   a. rarely, almost never.
   b. occasionally, mostly at certain times during the
      month.
   c. almost always.
5. Choose one word to describe your facial pores:
   a. microscopic.
   b. ordinary.
   c. craters.

To determine your skin type, look at your answers. If you
have mostly "a" answers, your skin is dry. A customized program will add needed moisture to your skin. If you circled
"b" most often, you are normal—isn't that a relief? A good
prevention plan will keep your skin looking as good in the
future as it does today. If the "c" showed up the most, you
have oily skin and probably know it. With some work and a
lot of knowledge, we can devise a regimen that will help you
love the face God gave you!

Dry Skin

Dry skin boasts small pores and no shine (a matte finish).
But expression lines form first on this type of skin, usually
around the eyes and lips, and on the forehead. When exposed
to the environment, dry skin becomes rough, flaky, and even
cracked. It rarely experiences blemishes but often feels tight
and dry. Dry skin tends to age faster than other skin types.

Cynthia Shares

As a beauty consultant who works with every skin type, I witness minor miracles. I've had clients drive out to my country house after several weeks of a successful treatment plan and exclaim in delight, "Look at my skin! Look at my skin!" Their happiness makes the effort worthwhile. Sometimes it takes a trial-and-error approach, as the client and I experiment with various skin-care programs and products. On the following pages, you'll find the basic skin-care plan I suggest for my clients.

Normal Skin

Normal skin does have visible pores, but not large, and the facial texture is relatively smooth. Neither dry nor oily, this type of skin often has a porcelain-doll quality. Lines and wrinkles will come later in life. In the meantime, blemishes usually don't pop up on this face, except perhaps when hormones are raging (as in menstruation or pregnancy).

Oily Skin

Oily skin produces too much oil—bottom line! The excessive oil gives this skin its telltale shine. It also clogs pores, causing blemishes, blackheads, and other unwanted bumps. With the extra oil production, pores get stretched and are usually quite large. Oily skin can even feel greasy or sticky to the touch. But the same oil that causes so much irritation will also keep this face young looking longer.

Combination Skin

Some women have combination skin with areas that are normal or dry, and a T-zone of oiliness. The T-zone consists of the forehead, nose, and chin. Shine will be evident here, and so will frequent breakouts. Products can control the oil production in the T-zone and add moisture to drier areas.

You can't change your skin type—the Serenity Prayer mentions accepting those things we can't alter. This is one of "those things." But you can change how you care for it, which will make the difference in your skin's appearance.

We have discovered that most skin problems are symptoms of a deeper internal problem. What goes in will most definitely come out . . . so, pure food in, lovely skin on the outside. Junk in, junky looking. Trust us, girls, garbage will eventually show up on the tip of your nose.

Beautiful skin is healthy skin. You may have noticed the pallor that comes over your countenance when you are sick. Your complexion is a reflection of your health, as are your other features like hair, nails, and figure.

We're firm believers in internal cleansing. Your skin is your largest organ, and it just happens to be one of your body's organs of elimination. Fasting is one way to speed the process of toxin elimination. So is dry-brushing: Take a loofah scrub and brush your entire body once a week before your bath or shower. Occasionally, we'll also do an internal cleanse. You can do intestinal cleanses, liver and kidney cleanses, even cleanses especially for your blood. Our books on health and nutrition, *The Healthy Balance* and *The Inner Balance*, will give you more information on cleanses and pure diets. You can also check our web site for information and ask at health food stores. To keep our skin looking its best, we eat lots of fruits and vegetables, including fresh vegetable juice, drink gallons of pure water, and avoid stress. And of course, we follow the skin-care plan outlined on the following pages.

Steps for Beautiful Skin

Let's design a skin-care program that will become a pleasant part of your daily beauty routine. Scientific research has shown that skin needs these five steps to stay healthy: cleanse, freshen, exfoliate, moisturize, and protect. These procedures benefit the four skin types we described above—dry, normal, oily, and combination. However, the products you choose for this system must be individualized. In the following pages, you'll learn the program and products that will work best for your own lovely complexion.

Cleanse

Consistent cleansing is the necessary first step of your skin-care program. Our faces are exposed to detrimental elements every day. City air is full of pollution and grime. In the country, we have dust and airborne crop particles. Add to that makeup, excess oil, and dead skin cells. No wonder our faces aren't as radiant as we would like! But creams and cleansers, used consistently, will soften while removing the soils that dull the surface of your skin.

Dry skin, because it doesn't have much natural oil and lubrication, needs a cleanser that removes impurities and dry, flaky skin cells without extracting any moisture. A cleansing cream, rich in emollients and oil, works best for this type of skin.

Normal and combination skin do best with light, water-soluble cleansers. You can cleanse with your fingertips or use a facecloth. This cleanser must remove cosmetics and other types of accumulation, plus excess oil in the T-zone. The cleansing routine below will work for dry, normal, and combination skin:

First, use an oil-free cosmetic remover to gently remove your makeup. Place the cleanser on your fingertips and lightly begin application. Start at the base of your neck and lightly stroke up and out. Cleanse your neck, then your chin and jawline. Think up, up, up—defy gravity! Move up to your mouth area with soft, circular motions and onto your cheeks and temples. Next smooth the product over your forehead, upward and outward, then down the bridge and sides of your nose. The eye area is last. Always use your ring finger to apply the lightest pressure to this delicate area. On your upper eyelid near the lashes, from the outside edge, stroke inward toward the nose, then sweep up below the eyebrow. Come around the eye and cleanse gently underneath, again sweeping inward toward the nose (see diagram).

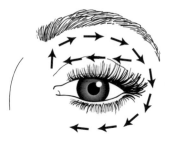

Never scrub or stretch your face while cleansing. This damages delicate tissues and can contribute to wrinkling. Instead, use your ring fingers to massage your skin gently. I (Cynthia) tense the muscles in the areas I'm working on. Remember isometrics? This seems to keep the skin of my face firm (or firmer, anyway). When asked about facial calisthenics, my dermatologist said that as long as you aren't causing wrinkles when you do them, they *might* help. If nothing else, exercise improves circulation above the neck in the same way it does below.

After application of your cleanser, use a damp washcloth to wipe it off. I (Cynthia) always splash with warm water after this step. I feel that if I haven't made a big, splashy mess when I'm cleaning, then I'm not thoroughly clean! My husband is thankful that I usually hop into the shower or bath for this. Don't use extremely warm or hot water on the face. It will only aggravate whatever your skin problems are. If it's dry, it will further strip valuable moisture from the skin. If it's oily, it will increase oil production. Instead, try comfortably warm water.

For dry and normal skin, a thorough cleansing every evening will probably suffice. Your skin will be clean and ready for moisture and other treatments before bed. In the morning, you can simply rinse with warm water to wake up.

Oily and combination skin, on the other hand, need extra cleansing sessions. Clean your skin at least twice a day, morning and night. Some women even need to sneak in a third cleansing in the middle of the day. Or you can blot the shine every few hours with lubricated facial cloths, especially created for this purpose.

Cleanse your oily skin with the same procedure used for normal skin. Your cleanser should be a liquid that foams when worked into a lather. Sudsy cleansers are best to strip your skin's oil and grime and buildup.

Exfoliate

You might think all this cleansing is enough to keep your skin fresh and radiant. Unfortunately, it's not. The cells of your epidermis are constantly being replaced. Dead cells accumulate. This is when you need to exfoliate—which means

Charity Chats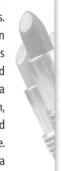

Models are always looking for inexpensive, easily available skin products. You can find some healthy exfoliants in your kitchen. Use oatmeal or corn meal to rub over your face before cleansing. Plain yogurt, which contains lactic acid, can be left on a clean face for twenty minutes and then removed with your cleanser and warm water. Gentle acids like these—lactic, alpha and beta hydroxyl, and fruit acids—exfoliate the skin, removing the rough, dry top layer. Years before, another beauty, the legendary Cleopatra, bathed in milk to keep her skin glowing and soothe away the desert sun's damage. Even then, she realized these mild acids were the wave of the future for a radiant, unforgettable complexion.

to take off or remove. So when you exfoliate your face, you are removing the top layer of dead skin cells. Exfoliants also stimulate the complexion, increasing circulation and bringing oxygen and nutrients to your skin. A biweekly mask is a great way to do all of this and pamper yourself at the same time.

Dry and normal skin benefit from a mildly abrasive mask with a creamy texture.

Combination and oily skin need masks that absorb excess sebum. Clay-based products lift off oil as they dry and harden on the skin. Very oily faces may need to exfoliate more often. I (Cynthia) have a client who uses her mask every morning in the shower. Her once-troubled skin is now gorgeous. Personally, we use a three-in-one product that contains cleanser, freshener, and exfoliant. We want to make wise use of our time. Besides, every night when we wash our faces, we're treated to facials! More about products like these on our web site and at the end of this book.

To exfoliate your skin, apply your mask of choice with light movements in the upward motions of the cleansing procedure. Avoid the eye and mouth areas. Leave your mask on for ten minutes, then soften with a warm washcloth. Remove gently and rinse well. Your face will look vibrant and alive.

Toner

Your toner, freshener, and/or astringent (the names of products for this next step) freshen the skin by removing any remaining residue. They tone and tighten your pores, giving your face a smoother, more refined appearance. The improved circulation results in a youthful radiance.

Choosing the right product for your skin is easy:

Dry and normal skin require a freshener that won't dry. Gentle liquids that contain botanicals will benefit your delicate skin. Avoid products with alcohol.

Combination and oily skin do well with a toner that "degreases" the surface of the skin. These industrial-strength products usually have alcohol as a main ingredient. This works well to deep-clean pores. The toner can be applied throughout the day to keep oil in check.

Using a cotton ball saturated with toner, apply in upward, outward motions (as you did with your cleanser), beginning at the neck. Freshen your entire face, avoiding the areas around the eyes and mouth.

Moisturize

Now your skin is ready for moisturizer and/or sunscreen. Moisturization is one of the most important steps of this program. Remember, moisture is the difference between a raisin and a grape! Healthy skin is nearly 90 percent water. Make sure you drink at least eight glasses of this essential liquid each day. But it's the oil in your skin, either natural or applied, that holds the water in the surface tissues to create lovely skin's soft suppleness. You need to find a balance in

Whatever type of moisturizer you choose, try this beauty secret that really works: Apply your lotion or cream on skin still slightly damp from a thorough cleansing. This locks the moisture into your skin. Moisturizer also conditions the texture of your skin and minimizes the appearance of fine, dry lines.

moisturizer formulas that fits your skin type perfectly. When you try a moisturizer, if more of the product stays on top of your skin rather than soaking in, it's probably too rich for you (or an inferior product).

Dry skin needs a moisturizer that's full of emollients. Apply to your entire face in an upward motion, but especially on dry areas like eyes, mouth, and neck. In the morning, use your moisturizer after cleansing and freshening. For a night cream, the richer, the better. Moisturizers containing lipids, humectants, and lubricants are available. Apply these liberally after cleansing to assure continued moisture for your thirsty skin.

Normal and combination skin types appreciate a lightweight moisturizer. Avoid the T-zone. Smooth on areas that feel tight and dry, and around eyes and mouth. Your neck also needs special attention. Eye creams are specially formulated to benefit areas of dry, thin, delicate skin.

Oily skin, believe it or not, can benefit from a moisturizer. After all, moisture is not oil, it's water! There are oil-free moisturizers available today. Check ingredients to find a light, water-based lotion. You will also want a moisturizer that's non-comedogenic, one that doesn't clog pores, resulting in pimples. For this skin type, only use moisturizer in the morning and evening on areas that become dehydrated: eyes, mouth, neck. The oil-free moisturizer will soften and smooth your skin.

Protect

To win a war, you must know your enemies. In the battle against time, your worst enemy is sunlight. We couldn't live without the sun. This gift from God does so much for our world. But its effects on our faces and bodies result in the wrinkles and blotches we are trying to avoid. Fortunately, we don't have to walk around hiding under parasols and bonnets anymore. Protective sunscreens are available for every skin type. Is one side of your face aging faster than the other? Usually it's the left side of your face. Can you guess why? Driving. While navigating your car every day, the left side of your face is taking a beating from the sun. Our friend Rosalyn says that the solution is to *not* apply sunscreen to the right side of your face until the damage equalizes itself! Our remedy is to wear more sunscreen—always—and dark glasses. You choose which one appeals to you!

All types of skin, no matter how dark, should use sunscreen. Aging skin isn't the only consequence of too much sun; a variety of cancers are also common. Look for products that contain ingredients to screen out the rays of UVA (that cause aging of the skin) and UVB (that burn) with an SPF (sun protection factor) of at least 15. Many moisturizers and some foundations now contain sunscreen. If you decide on one of these, you'll eliminate a beauty step. For oily skin, try a water-based product. And don't forget to protect your eyes and the surrounding area by always wearing sunglasses when outdoors.

As a model, I (Charity) am often called to do a beachwear shoot with only a few days' notice. I'm supposed to show up camera-ready with a savage tan. How does a blue-eyed, blonde, Irish girl live up to such tough expectations? Self-tanner! I refuse to bake my skin in the sun. Not only do self-tanners darken skin without damage by UV rays, they nourish with

A Model's Monthly Facial

Boil water in a deep pot. You can add herbs for a fresh scent. Hold a towel over your head, like a tent, and steam your face for five to ten minutes. This will open your clogged pores, releasing oil, grime, and toxins.

Next, use a sudsy cleanser with warm water.

After you rinse, you can use one of the masks mentioned. Mud masks and mint masks are also nice.

Rinse off well. Pat dry. Use your freshener and reapply your moisturizer. Enjoy your new skin—it's almost a miracle!

aloe, vitamin E, and other added moisturizers. Don't be afraid to try them. Self-tanners have improved over the years. They no longer leave you a streaked, tangerine orange like they used to.

For best results with a self-tanner, exfoliate your skin first—through shaving, or with a loofah or rough washcloth. Then smear on body lotion liberally. This helps the tanner spread evenly. Apply over areas you want tanned. You can reapply for a darker tan, but only cover elbows, knees, and ankles once, or they'll be darker than the rest of your body. Several hours later, you're ready for the beach!

Now you have the five steps to healthy skin. This is a program that, once learned, takes very little time. Yet it yields numerous beauty benefits. Make it a part of your daily routine, and your radiant complexion will be the talk of the town. Even more important is your inner glow. Scripture gives us instructions for this vital area.

Soul Surgery

In Scripture, our spiritual skin is called the flesh. The word implies weakness, frailty, imperfections (both physical and moral); sinfulness and tendencies to sin; carnal nature, seat of carnal appetites and desires (wanting to satisfy them); sinful passions and affections; and our wills and self-centeredness.[1] Biblical examples of the flesh in Galatians 5:19–21 would be sexual sins of every kind, gluttony and drunkenness, strife, temper, competitiveness, greed, willfulness, selfishness, and so on.

Over time, we can accumulate too much flesh physically, on our faces or bodies. The excess becomes obvious. We notice it in the mirror. Everyone else can see it too. A surgeon might suggest cutting off the excess, whether it's warts or wrinkles we're removing. In like manner, when we operate in our spiritual flesh, the mirror of God's Word exposes it. Others become painfully aware of our condition. The Great Physician has his way of cutting off our excess spiritual flesh. He uses the sharp two-edged sword of Scripture to trim it away. He also employs circumstances and other people.

> "Some women
> are not beautiful—
> they only look as though
> they are."
>
> —writer Karl Kraus

Just as we all desire healthy skin for our faces, so we want healthy spiritual skin. Leprosy is a disease that eats away the flesh and tissues of the face and body. There is a leprosy that can affect our spiritual skin—it's called bitterness. Hebrews 12:15 warns us: "See to it that no one comes short of the grace of God; that no root of bitterness springing up causes trouble, and by it many be defiled."

When we hang on to hurts and emotional bumps and bruises, when we nurture our grievances and don't forgive, bitterness develops, marring the grace and beauty that we have in Christ. But when we forgive, our emotional wounds are freed up to heal completely. We then have the liberty of spirit to reach out to others in the warmth and genuine love of Jesus Christ.

Several years ago, I (Cynthia) was tested in this very area while teaching a large Bible study in our town. Every week one woman (we'll call her Beulah) attended with the intent of destroying my reputation and the class. Throughout the lesson, she would make derogatory remarks about me and my teaching to those around her. Beulah prided herself in devising questions and dilemmas to trip me up (or attempt to do so). She blurted them out at classes. Beulah stirred up those around her each Wednesday, disrupted the class with her outbursts, and then slandered me the rest of the week. She even complained to the pastor about me.

Each time Beulah asked her accusatory questions in class, I would answer her with a searched-out explanation, offered in love. Others in the class verified that Beulah was always treated with compassion. But by the end of the three-month study, I was fed up with Beulah. I didn't have very nice feelings toward her and was in emotional turmoil about the experience. I prayed, "Lord, don't allow me to become bitter. Give me an opportunity to redeem this situation."

And he did. But not the way I would have chosen. I would have preferred that God intervene in his powerful way—you know, sent some lightning or something. A direct hit over Beulah's house! But instead, he humbled me. Beulah started her own Bible study, and the Lord put it on my heart to be one of her students. I attended the little group faithfully each week, sat right next to my enemy, flooded her with praise, asked her for advice, sent encouraging notes, prayed for her. I was so sweet over those several months it almost made me cry!

And God did a work. Not only in my heart but in Beulah's as well. She warmed up. Began talking to me like a human being. Even gave me a hug now and then. These days, Beulah wants to be best friends. Through that experience, I learned that Jesus Christ is the Redeemer. He can redeem *any* situation. Not only does he save our souls from hell, he can restore relationships that we might write off forever.

When we allow our flesh to indulge in bitterness (which we sometimes savor when someone has truly hurt us), we hinder God's redeeming power in our lives and those around us. I could have "defiled" so many with my venom against that woman. Because I refused to become bitter, I remained the gracious woman that I want to be as a witness for Christ.

Leprosy is caused by a bacteria. From ages past, it has been considered to be very contagious. Leviticus 13 gives advice for dealing with leprous people: Put them out of the midst of the congregation. Don't have any part of them. Likewise, be careful of those with leprous spirits. Don't let their bitterness influence our church gatherings, family unity, harmony among friends. The Bible's advice of putting them out of our midst might be most appropriate. Stay away from bitter people! Bitterness is highly contagious!

I (Charity) have discovered that we wear our spiritual status on our faces. As I have traveled the States as a speaker and singer, I've met so many women. The ones who have spent years living in bitterness show it on their faces. Hard, tight lips, angry eyes. Worry shows up on a face with lines and a fearful expression. Those who are still insecure with low self-worth and don't yet enjoy the unconditional love of the Savior reflect that in their appearance. Those who are in the Word and are experiencing the love of the Lord and his joy and peace show that too. No matter their age, they radiate their inner beauty. They are a joy to be around!

Second Chances

Thankfully, God gives people of flesh second (and at times, third, fourth, and even more) chances. His very nature is full of mercy. The story of Moses in Exodus 32 demonstrates this compassion. Moses had gone up Mount Sinai to receive the tablets with God's commandments and the instructions for building the tabernacle. But his time with the Lord was cut short when God told Moses to go down the mountain at once, because the people had corrupted themselves with idolatry. God threatened to destroy the people and start over with Moses, but Moses interceded for the people and for the honor of the Lord's name.

With that crisis past, Moses hustled down the mountain, the Ten Commandments in hand, and witnessed God's people worshiping the golden calf. He became so angry that he smashed the Ten Commandments, newly written by the very finger of God. (Remember, Moses had some trouble with his temper before. Way back in Egypt he had killed the Egyptian who whipped the Jewish slave.)

But in Exodus 34, Moses is commanded to head back up the mountain to receive the Commandments a second time. God demonstrated mercy to the people, saying, "Cut out for yourself two stone tablets *like the former ones,* and I will write on the tablets the words that were on the former tablets *which you shattered*" (v. 1, emphasis ours). In spite of this angry action (which God reminded him of), the Lord gave Moses and the people a second chance. This time around God showed his servant more than mercy—he showed him his glory.

Yes, the Lord has grace for the sin and weakness of men and women, as demonstrated by the life of Moses. But if we don't curb our flesh, God eventually will. Moses continued to struggle with his temper at times, often (understandably) irritated by the children of Israel. As they journeyed through the wilderness, the Israelites sometimes couldn't find drinking water. They complained quite loudly to Moses. Once before, God had commanded Moses to strike a rock and watch life-giving water flow out. The second time, however, God told Moses to simply speak to the rock. Instead of obeying, the frustrated leader got mad and struck it again. The consequence of Moses' fleshly action was that he would not be permitted his one desire, to enter the Promised Land.

A Secret for Conquering the Flesh

In the Old Testament, believers sacrificed the flesh of an animal to pay for their sins. This was a foreshadowing of what was to come. In the New Testament, Jesus' sacrifice on the cross paid the price of sin once and for all. Because of this, we sacrifice our flesh on a daily basis when we surrender to his lordship. This is the new covenant that Christ brought to his people. This is our salvation.

> **"This is hope in a jar."**
>
> —Charles Revson, founder of Revlon Cosmetics, introducing his revolutionary skin cream in 1958

In the Old Testament, the law was given to control the old nature, the flesh. After Pentecost, the Holy Spirit was sent to control the flesh. When we submit to the Holy Spirit on a daily (even momentary) basis, our flesh is crucified and we become more like Christ. This is our sanctification.

> **"This is hope in a book."**
>
> —Cynthia and Charity on their book on the eternal beauty of godliness

The Holy Spirit is our secret weapon as Christians for conquering our old nature, or fleshly will and appetites. Scripture says that the flesh profits nothing. The apostle Paul wrote that in his flesh, there was no good thing (Rom. 7:18). When Jesus spoke to Nicodemus one night (John 3), he explained that we are all born of the flesh but must be born again of the Spirit. There is hope.

Romans 8:1–2 reminds us that "there is now no condemnation for those who are in Christ Jesus. For the law of the Spirit of life in Christ Jesus has set you free from the law of sin and of death."

As we close, let's use the steps for healthy physical skin to get healthy spiritually.

- *Cleanse* by the washing of the Word: "that He might sanctify her [the church], having cleansed her by the washing of water with the word" (Eph. 5:26). Clean up your act. Seek forgiveness. Get into Scripture and stay there!

- *Freshen* with the fellowship of believers: "But if we walk in the Light as He Himself is in the Light, we have fellowship with one another, and the blood of Jesus His Son cleanses us from all sin" (1 John 1:7). Iron sharpens iron, Scripture says (Prov. 27:17). In Philippians 2:2, Paul asked that his joy be made complete by the church having "the same mind, maintaining the same love, united in spirit, intent on one purpose." Other believers challenge, inspire, admonish, and comfort us. We need each other. Stay connected!

- *Exfoliate* by submitting to God and others. Remember you are a diamond in the rough. The Lord uses circumstances (trials and tribulations especially) to polish off the sharp edges. He also employs people in the process—husbands and wives, authorities in our lives, strong-willed children or mothers-in-law, or the Beulahs of the world. "For we are the true circumcision, who worship in the Spirit of God and glory in Christ Jesus and put no confidence in the flesh" (Phil. 3:3).

- *Moisturize* with the oil of the Holy Spirit. Just as your parched physical skin craves moisture, so your spirit thirsts for the filling of the Holy Spirit. Jesus said in John 7, "'If anyone is thirsty, let him come to Me and drink. He who believes in Me, as the Scripture said, "From his innermost being will flow rivers of living water."' But this He spoke of the Holy Spirit" (vv. 37–39). The indwelling Spirit is God's answer for godly living here on earth. And he is the seal of our salvation for eternity. Oil has always symbolized God's Spirit. Scripture speaks of the oil of gladness. If moisture is the difference between a plum and a prune, then the Spirit is the difference between a joy-filled believer and a prune-faced Christian.

- *Protect* because we have an enemy who is out to steal from us and even destroy our lives. His name is Satan, and 1 Peter 5:8 calls him a roaring lion, who prowls about looking for someone to devour. He's a formidable force, a devious liar. But God is greater—and he is in us! Hebrews 2:14 assures us that Christ himself partook of flesh and blood so that "through death He might render powerless him who had the power of death, that is, the devil." The Lord has provided sure protection from the devil. James tells us to resist him. We can oppose our enemy, standing firm against his schemes, by putting on the full armor of God, as outlined in Ephesians 6:12–17:

For our struggle is not against flesh and blood, but against the rulers, against the powers, against the world forces of this darkness, against the spiritual forces of wickedness in the heavenly places. Therefore, take up the full armor of God, that you may be able to resist in the evil day, and having done everything, to stand firm. Stand firm therefore, having girded your loins with truth, and having put on the breastplate of righteousness, and having shod your feet with the preparation of the gospel of peace; in addition to all, taking up the shield of faith with which you will be able to extinguish all the flaming arrows of the evil one. And take the helmet of salvation, and the sword of the Spirit, which is the word of God.

Top Beauty Secret

Now you have a plan for physical and spiritual beauty. Are you excited about the program? Do you hope these special treatments will give your face a new luster? Want to know how to really shine? Spend time with Jesus Christ. That's right. Time spent with God will give you a radiance that others will ask about. You'll have to inform them, "It can't be bought in a bottle." Only the Lord himself can provide this kind of glow!

Remember when Moses climbed back up Mount Sinai to receive a second set of the Ten Commandments? Exodus 34:29 says that his face shone because he had seen God's glory. When he returned down the mountain, his face gleamed so brightly that the Israelites were afraid of him. Moses had to cover the radiance with a veil!

Have you felt energized and invigorated after spending a glorious time with the Lord, either alone or in group worship? Our faces reflect the spirit of Christ within us. Shining, clear eyes. Glowing, joyful faces. Beautiful, genuine smiles. Yes, a makeover miracle!

5 | The Windows of Your Soul

When talking with a friend, what are her two facial features that stand out to you most? Doesn't your gaze usually focus on her eyes and her smile? Eyes and lips are the most expressive features we possess. They deserve chapters all their own: eyes in this one, lips in the next.

Your eyes. Big or small, blue, brown, or green. They express what's going on in your soul. Women can force a huge smile onto their lips. But their eyes betray what's in their hearts.

We talk with our eyes. Ask any child. They can read their parents' thoughts through glances, stares, and other expressions. Cynthia's mother only had to frown at her children, and it was more effective than a paddling. (Or maybe we knew that was next!) We all express our emotions with our eyes. Can't you tell by looking in your husband's eyes whether he's feeling sympathy or anger after your little fender bender? Even though your son's words are brave before his big game, does his expression reveal some fear? When your daughter's heart is broken, can you see the hurt in her eyes?

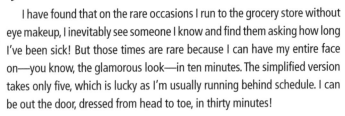

Cynthia Shares

I have found that on the rare occasions I run to the grocery store without eye makeup, I inevitably see someone I know and find them asking how long I've been sick! But those times are rare because I can have my entire face on—you know, the glamorous look—in ten minutes. The simplified version takes only five, which is lucky as I'm usually running behind schedule. I can be out the door, dressed from head to toe, in thirty minutes!

Eyes truly are the windows to our souls. Through them, others can see the emotions bubbling just below the surface. Our eyes radiate our joy, reveal our sadness, and flash fire when we're mad. And of course, we view the world through these ocular windows. Because our eyes are so important, they deserve special care. We wouldn't want to live without them, would you?

Making Eyes

Eyes are also one of the most important features on your face. These beauty assets stand out when enhanced with well-applied cosmetics. Many women feel that their eyes fade into their face without some mascara and liner. They wouldn't leave the house without either. And since eyes are most important, we need to make them up first. Once when I (Charity) was being driven hurriedly to a meeting, I started my makeup with my mouth. Before working all the way up to my eyes, we were at the appointment and I ended up meeting business prospects with a bold "I Love Lucy" mouth and naked eyes. Scary!

Applying cosmetics should never take very long. If it did, most of us wouldn't bother with it—we have more important things to do! The secret lies in practice and a good routine. If

Eye Openers

Start your day with a glass of fresh-squeezed orange or carrot juice. Vitamins C and A are powerful antioxidants, vitamins that protect your valuable vision. (You can find more nutrition tips in our next book, *The Healthy Balance.*)

Be sure to rest your eyes while reading, working on the computer, or doing hand work. Keep from straining.

Always wear sunglasses. UVB rays can damage the retina as well as the skin's collagen.

Oil-free eye makeup remover will remove cosmetics without leaving a filmy residue on your eyes.

If you have a disease that affects the eyes, like diabetes or glaucoma, or you're on medication that affects the eyes, get regular medical checkups. Follow your doctor's orders explicitly. Your eyesight is too precious to lose!

you're new at makeup application, don't give up. Remember the old adage, practice makes perfect. And you'll look practically perfect if you keep at it. Day by day, your skill will eventually rival a Hollywood pro. Your routine, the order that you do each cosmetic step, allows you to put your makeup on without thinking. You know that favorite recipe that you make almost weekly, the one that you can throw together while chatting on the phone with a friend? Even the pickiest eater raves about that dish when you serve it. Well, that's how easy this recipe for looking good becomes with practice—and then, *you'll* be all the rave!

Highbrow Eyebrows

Since your brows frame your eyes, let's start there.

There's nothing worse than caterpillar brows. Once a teenage girl came into the salon where I (Cynthia) worked asking for a wax job. I was untrained in such things, but my boss insisted. I carefully applied the wax, and then, rip! Off went the brow—and some of the young woman's forehead too! But she still tipped me well and called me her "hero," because there's nothing worse than caterpillar brows!

Have your brows professionally shaped with tweezers or wax—by someone with experience! Or tweeze them yourself. First, brush eyebrows straight up, then smooth just the upper hairs of your brows. This will outline their arch and natural shape. You can design a more pleasing shape using an eye pencil.

Line up the pencil vertically alongside your nose, as in the diagram (1). This is where the inside corner of your brow should begin. You can mark this spot with a soft eyeliner pencil.

Next, line the pencil from your nostril to the outside of your eye (2). Your brow should end here. Mark this area too.

Hold the pencil parallel to your eye across the bridge of your nose, touching the inner and outer ends of your brows (3). Your brows should begin and end at about the same level—or the brow can have a slight lift at the end, if you prefer.

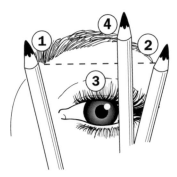

Last, place the pencil vertically along the outside edge of the iris of your eye (4). The point in your eyebrow where the pencil intersects should be the highest point of your arch.

Mark this point. You can draw a desirable shape with the soft eye pencil. Tweeze all stray hairs that fall outside this shape, between your eyes, under your arch, at your temple, on your forehead. Leave the upper edge of your natural brows alone. Do not overtweeze.

Shape both brows. With a tiny comb or toothbrush designated for this purpose, comb your brows up again. If they are too long, trim with scissors. Comb them into shape. Fill in any bare spots with brow pencil in a shade similar to your hair color or slightly darker, if light blonde. Black pencil is too severe. Draw soft, tiny strokes, then brush, blending the color into your natural brows. Well-shaped brows give a professional, classy appearance.

Here are a few tips Charity has learned while modeling:

- If brows tend to grow wild, comb them into shape, first spraying a little hairspray (gel or mousse work too) on the comb or brush. (Or brow tamers are available at your nearest drugstore.)
- Got a low pain tolerance? Deaden the brow area with ice for fifteen seconds before you begin to tweeze hairs.
- Use the correct terminology. We tweeze a brow—we pluck a turkey!
- Create a nice full shape, but don't remove excessively. Take your time and tweeze strategically.
- And remember, no unibrows!

Lining Things Up

If you only have a minute or two for makeup, eyeliner is an important step. The liner defines your eyes, accenting their shape, drawing your eyes out of hiding. Liquid liner goes in and out of fashion. If you decide to use it, have a steady hand and draw a thin line at the base of your lashes. Personally, we like creamy eyeliner pencils. They go on smooth and easy and look more natural than other forms of liner.

You want a pencil soft enough that it doesn't pull on your delicate eyelids—but not so soft that it breaks with each use. (To firm it up, leave it in the refrigerator overnight. This works with soft lipsticks too.) Eye pencils that automatically self-sharpen are available now. They tend to be blunter than the old-fashioned pencil you can sharpen with a metal sharpener. Decide what works for you.

The eye pencil shade you choose depends on your complexion and hair coloring. Black can be harsh unless you are very dark. More flattering shades are charcoal, dark gray, and even navy. Sable brown looks great on women with warm coloring: brown hair and brown eyes, blondes and redheads with golden complexions. And then there are fun colors for evening: shimmering blues, greens, plum, and even silver and gold.

We only recommend eyeliner at your upper lash line if you have a good amount of upper eyelid. If not, the dark line at the top of the eye tends to do the opposite of what's desired. Unless the line is very thin (an extension of the lashes) it may close up the eye area and make it look heavy and small. The line also emphasizes any lid overhang you might have—bad for us as we age. Cynthia doesn't wear upper eyeliner, unless that's all the eye makeup she's wearing that day.

If you do wear upper eyeliner, begin a tapered line between the inner corner and iris of the eye. Liner and shadows close to the nose make your eyes appear too close-set and draw attention to your nose. Is this the effect you're after? Not us! Make soft strokes as close to the lash line as possible. End at the edge of your eyes, or slightly beyond. Extending liner into the temple area went out with Cleopatra!

Most eyes benefit from a line under lower lashes. Starting at the outside, lower edge of the eye (but not intersecting with an upper line, which makes the eye look smaller), make light, soft strokes (like an artist's) close to the base of your lower lashes. Never make a hard, thick line. Again, you want to taper off just to the inside edge of the iris, leaving a little space between your iris and the inner corner of your eye. Liner, top and bottom, should start and stop where your natural lashes do. You can smudge this line with a cosmetic applicator or cotton swab for a natural, smoky effect.

We highly recommend the use of Q-tips while making up. The proper use of this favorite makeup tool can make the difference between the "painted on" look and clean, natural-looking eye makeup. So, buy yourself a box of them, and blend, blend, blend!

You can redefine your eyes with liner. For close-set eyes, line only the outer half of upper and lower lids. You can even extend past the eyes a little. To elongate round eyes, increase the thickness of the line as you draw, thin on the inner lid, thicker on the outside. For very small eyes, create a soft line just under the iris of the eye and not as close to the lash line. This seems to round out and open up the eyes. Small eyes also appear larger when lined with a dark eye shadow. Load a thin, fine brush with the powder and smooth it close to upper and lower lashes.

Out from the Shadows

Eye shadow definitely adds glamour to your appearance. You may decide against eye shadow for daytime wear, sticking with mascara and liner to give your eyes emphasis. The only shadow Cynthia wears by day is a charcoal shade brushed

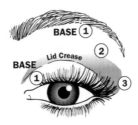

along the crease. This creates the illusion of a natural shadowy contour. Daytime shadows should be subtle and natural—grays, browns, taupes, navy blues, lavender grays, etc., preferably without sparkles. This gives a professional polish, but doesn't scream, "I'm wearing makeup!"

For evening, you can get away with more intense color, shimmer, and shine. Neutrals and colors come in several forms: pressed powder shadows that can be applied wet or dry, creme formulas in cake or stick forms, and creme-to-powder formulas that smooth on like a creme but dry to a powder with staying power.

First, using a sponge applicator or brush, apply a light or bright color as a base from the lash line up to the brow (1). This provides a smooth surface to grab your contour shade.

For contouring, choose deeper colors, shades that look like your eyes' natural shadows. This makeup trick works best with eyes wide open. See the crease of your eyelid? You are going to shade this area with darker color. At the crease and just above, stroke on color with a brush or applicator, beginning at the outer edge of each eye, working in toward nose (2). Remember, stop short of the inner corner of the eye.

Take your brush and wedge some color at the outer edge down to the lash line (3). Don't stop there. With another brush or fingertip, blend, blend, blend the two shadows together and the outside edges of the shading.

If you end up buying an eye shadow that's too intense, you can tone it down by sweeping an ivory-colored matte shadow over the top. Blending is a must with all your shadows. Buy a professional eye shadow brush and use it. Powder your lids first to remove excess oils, then shadow. This will make blending easier.

Lash but Not Least

We leave the most important step for last: mascara. In a national survey, this lash-lengthening, eye-opening cosmetic was voted the Big Gun in most women's beauty artillery. If you only have time for one makeup procedure, this is it. Mascara comes in many formulas: thickening to coat each lash, lengthening that actually contains fibers to make lashes appear longer, conditioning with vitamins to add shine, and waterproof for days at the beach or when you're expecting a good cry. Whatever type you buy, make sure to change mascara every three months to avoid bacteria contamination. And remember not to pump your wand before you apply your mascara—that only pumps air into the container, drying the product out quicker. Instead, swirl the wand around, gathering mascara from the sides of the tube.

Starting with the first eye, apply mascara to the tips of your lashes, holding the wand vertically. Next, apply mascara to the base of the lashes and curving up and out. Be sure to color the lashes on the outside edges of your eye. Hold the wand vertically again and brush color on your lower lashes, one at a time. Using an eyelash curler before or after mascara will open up the eyes even further. Cynthia curls just after the first step of darkening the tips of her lashes. Then top off with another quick coat. Makeup artists comb through before this second application.

Charity powders her lashes before applying makeup. This gives the mascara a little something more to hang on to.

Then—here's a great trick for you—she holds her eyelash curler against a heated curling iron for just three seconds, waits one second, and then curls. The heated curler curls the lashes much faster and the curl lasts longer. But remember, it only has to be warm to work, not hot. Next, apply coats of black mascara, and do the other eye. Voilà, heartbreaker eyes! (Mop up any mistakes with a damp cotton swab. Mistakes can be a distraction to the beholder.)

Two women with sparkling eyes:

Catherine Booth, founder of the Salvation Army, read the Bible through eight times by the time she was twelve years old. **Susanna Wesley**, mother of many offspring (nearly twenty!) fed herself and her children on the Word daily. Her two sons, Charles and John Wesley, founded the Methodist denomination and wrote many great hymns of the faith.

Inner Eyelights

When you have completed your makeup, enhancing your eyes, others are attracted to gaze into these windows. In doing so, they get a glimpse into your soul. Even strangers will be attracted to the light in your eyes and want to know where it comes from.

In Luke 11:34–35, Jesus talked about our eyes. "The eye is the lamp of your body," he said. "When your eye is clear, your whole body also is full of light; but when it is bad, your body also is full of darkness. Then watch out that the light in you is not darkness."

Do you understand what the Lord is talking about? Surely you do. I (Cynthia) watched a heavy metal band on television. Their eyes were dark, empty, at times even full of evil and hatred. The windows to their souls revealed a spiritual bankruptcy that was painful to see.

We witnessed this in a young woman we led to Christ. Before receiving the Lord, Danine practiced witchcraft. Her eyes were dark and dull. There was no sparkle in them, no life. Involvement with Satan's world means death, and that's what Danine's eyes revealed. But after Christ came into her heart, a transformation took place. Her eyes reflected the Lord's light and life. They twinkled when she smiled, which she did continually.

Satan can use the garbage we take in to get a hook into our very souls. As we have traveled the country, we've heard this story repeatedly with different names, different situations:

- "My husband enjoyed watching R-rated movies. Next thing I knew, he brought home some X-rated films. He got hooked on pornography and ran off with another woman."
- "My daughter stayed in her room for hours listening to heavy-metal rock music. She began to hang around with a bad crowd and soon was doing drugs with them."
- "I found *Playboy* magazines under my fourteen-year-old son's bed. What should I do?"
- "My best friend constantly reads romance novels filled with explicit sex scenes. She began an Internet romance, eventually running off with the guy, leaving her husband and three children behind."

Stories like these are commonplace today because we are feeding our minds pollution. With it, Satan tempts us and leads us into sin. Our eyes are one vehicle. The same is true with our other senses: our hearing, touch, taste, and even smell. We live in a very sensual society. God made us with keen senses, and he desires that we use these gifts. But we are to use them appropriately, in the right timing, to serve him.

Cynthia Shares

According to Jesus, the eyes are the lamps of the body. He also says that our eyes should be clear. While shopping in Wal-Mart one day, I understood the full meaning of Jesus' words. I was walking down the aisle with a cart, and two children—a boy and a girl, around ten years old—came strolling toward me. I looked into their eyes and saw innocence, clarity, and yes, light. These days we can see darkness even in the eyes of young children. They are jaded and worldly wise. Their innocence has been lost. They are already burdened by sin; if not by experience, then by the knowledge of it. But these children were different. Not a word was exchanged, but I thought, "I wonder if these are Christian kids?"

In a moment, my question was answered. Behind them came their Amish mother, hurrying to catch up with her offspring. These children had obviously been shielded from the corruption that so many are exposed to these days, which floods in through eye-gates and degrades souls. Our children lose their innocence, and we lose our sensitivity to sin. We must protect what we allow our eyes to see. Our minds are like computers, and our eyes are the entry system. What we see, our minds catalog away for future reference. The evil we take in is never fully erased.

Unfortunately, the sensuality of our day is often connected to immorality. We must be careful what we allow into our lives through our eyes and ears. Cynthia often warns her kids, "You wouldn't eat garbage, so don't put it into your minds."

Remember the three little monkeys, See No Evil, Hear No Evil, Speak No Evil? Can't you see those cute little critters now, their hands covering their eyes, ears, and mouth? They weren't about to let evil enter their thoughts and then come back out. What goes into our minds will sneak out eventually. The Book of Proverbs assures us of this: "For as he thinks within himself, so he is" (23:7). It's just a matter of time before we're saying and doing the things we've witnessed on television, in movies, on the Internet, in books and magazines, or through music. And the darkness is expressed through our eyes.

A few years ago, we were mentoring a wonderful young man who wanted to go into the ministry. As Doug (not his real name) grew close to the Savior, he was joyful and full of light. Later, though, he chose to become sexually involved with a young married woman. Then Doug's eyes were dark and depressed. A breach quickly developed in our once-close friendship. After much prayer and counseling, the prodigal son went forward in church, repenting of the sinful relationship. Doug was again full of joy and restored to fellowship with his Lord and God's people. As he hugged those of us who had followed him to the altar, his eyes reflected the joy and light of complete forgiveness.

First John 1:7 tells us that "if we walk in the Light as He Himself is in the Light, we have fellowship one with another, and

> **Tropicana Orange Juice:** "Satisfy a deeper thirst."
>
> **Jesus Christ:** Satisfy a deeper thirst—"If anyone is thirsty, let him come to Me and drink. He who believes in Me, as the Scripture said, 'From his innermost being will flow rivers of living water.' . . . Whoever drinks of the water that I will give him shall never thirst; but the water that I will give him will become in him a well of water springing up to eternal life" (John 7:37–38; 4:13–14).

the blood of Jesus His Son cleanses us from all sin." When we receive Jesus as our Savior, we experience the washing away of our sins. We know true, unconditional love for the first time. The darkness is gone; the light floods in. Unconfessed sin casts a shadow over this relationship. We must "walk as children of light . . . trying to learn what is pleasing to the Lord" (Eph. 5:8,10).

Cynthia Shares

When people ask about the victories in my life, I have to point to this one habit that I've developed: I take in as much of the Word as I possibly can. I can honestly say that I'm now addicted to consumption of Scripture.

What's your addiction? Is there something you've just got to have? Coffee, Coke, candy? Psalm 19:10 says that God's commandments are "sweeter also than honey and the drippings of the honeycomb." The psalmist exclaims to the Lord in Psalm 119:103: "How sweet are Your words to my taste! Yes, sweeter than honey to my mouth!" Due to health problems, I can't eat anything sweet. Instead, God's Word is my sugar—I can't live without it!

I have times in my life, however, when I get too busy. I don't spend as much time in the Word. You know the old saying, "If the devil can't get you bad, he'll get you busy." This is so true of my life. Charity admits it too. How about you? Do trivial matters seem to drown out the really important things in your life? I have to continually evaluate how I'm spending my time. If my biblical priorities—God first, family second, other commitments third—are out of balance, then I correct my schedule, weeding out the nonessentials.

I'd like to share with you my plan for Scripture intake. This program has provided me with a deep relationship with Jesus Christ, a growing knowledge of God, his Word and his ways, correction of sinful attitudes and actions in my life, transformed character, faith to trust that a big God can produce big dreams in my life, faith to continue trusting when the storms come, and a love for others with concern for their eternal welfare. Try it, and see what it does for you!

Want to know how you can have and keep this beautiful light in your eyes? The secret is found in Psalm 19:8: "The commandment of the Lord is pure, *enlightening* the eyes" (emphasis ours).

To illuminate our minds and souls, programming them with good instead of bad, we must take in as much of God's

Word as possible. We spend so much time filling our minds with the world's propaganda. How much time do we take to nurture our spirits with truth? Not much, according to various polls. For example, in a recent survey of seminary students (young men and women preparing for full-time Christian ministry), most of those interviewed admitted that they don't have regular devotional times.

But let's get up close and personal. How much time do you spend in God's Word? As sisters in Christ, we encourage you to make a fresh commitment, here and now, to devote some time each day to Bible intake.

Cynthia's Personal "Inner Beauty" Routine

Through spiritual disciplines, I (Cynthia) attempt to absorb truth through every avenue available, even through my senses. I take in spiritual truth through my eyes, ears, mind, heart, and even voice. Did you know that you can experience God's Word in body and soul? Read on.

With my eyes, I read the Word daily. I may be working through a book of the Bible or participating in a "read the Bible in a year" program. Another plan offers a schedule of an Old Testament passage, a New Testament passage, a Psalm, and several Proverbs each day. Like me, you might enjoy one of the modern translations for your reading: the New King James, the New Living Translation, or even a paraphrase like the Living Bible.

This is not study. It's simply getting into God's Word and enjoying it. Allowing your God to speak to your spirit. Allowing Scripture to sweep into your heart and soul, refreshing and renewing you. Reading can be long or short, depending on the time available that day. And I always (with only emergencies as exceptions) read Scripture daily to my kids.

We call it "Bible and Breakfast." This practice has paid off big-time in the lives of my five children, who all love and serve the Lord.

Another way to take in Scripture with your eyes is to place Scripture verses around your house—posters, wall hangings, even refrigerator magnets. The Internet is another modern tool. You and your family can continually expose your eyes (and your hearts) to the truth.

Deuteronomy 6:6–9 instructs us to train our children this way:

> These words, which I am commanding you today, shall be on your heart. You shall teach them diligently to your sons and shall talk of them when you sit in your house and when you walk by the way and when you lie down and when you rise up. You shall bind them as a sign on your hand and they shall be as frontals on your forehead. You shall write them on the doorposts of your house and on your gates.

Some eyes are blind to spiritual things. We need to pray for each other continually that the Holy Spirit will remove the blinders Satan has placed over some spiritual eyes, that the dear one will see truth and respond positively.

With my ears, I hear God's Word. Scripture says that the person who hears truth is blessed. I have been blessed through the practice of listening to God's Word (via cassette tapes) as I go about my day. When I'm doing housework, ironing, or cooking family meals, I carry my cassette player along and plug into the Word. I'm in such a habit now and love listening so much that I feel lost without the sound of Scripture in the background. I have gone through the complete Bible several times, studying it verse by verse with Dr. J. Vernon McGee's delightful Thru the Bible course. I've also listened through the Old and New Testaments as I've washed dishes and scrubbed floors. Some of the taped sets even have music and dramatization. If I'm alone in the car, I'll sometimes listen there. More often, I pray or work on memorizing verses. If I'm chauffeuring the kids, I use the time to build relationships with them or talk about some important issues. In the car, they are my captive audience!

When I've listened through the entire Bible for another time, I'll often take a break and listen to one of my favorite Bible preachers. Atlanta pastor Charles Stanley has influenced my spiritual life more than anyone else. Occasionally, I'll listen to radio preachers and teachers. I also listen to Scripture-based songs and sing along.

But it's the Scriptures themselves that satisfy my soul and renew my mind like nothing else. The continual hearing of God's Word really does transform our thinking, as Romans 12:2 promises: "Be transformed by the renewing of your mind, so that you may prove what the will of God is, that which is good and acceptable and perfect."

Immersing ourselves in Scripture also produces the peace Paul spoke of in Philippians 4:8–9: "Whatever is true, whatever is honorable, whatever is right, whatever is pure, whatever is lovely, whatever is of good repute, if there is any excellence and if anything worthy of praise, dwell on these things. . . . And the God of peace will be with you."

What could be more excellent and worthy of praise than God's own Word? Do you have trouble with negative, critical thoughts about yourself or others? I confess that I was this way until I began listening to God's Word constantly. I would be doing dishes after church, and my thoughts would wander: *What an awful job I did on the piano offertory this morning during worship! I should have practiced more. Why do I even bother? I'm just not good enough . . . Why didn't Jan talk to me today after service? She'd better not be mad because Ana invited me to ride to the retreat with her. That upsets me! Ana can invite who she wants to ride with her. I saw Jan whispering to Mary over in the corner by the women's restroom. They were probably talking about Ana and me. That hurts my feelings . . .*

Seriously, at times stupid thoughts like these would cycle through my thinking. My husband calls it my "wild imagination." Scripture calls it "vain imaginings." To rein in these fantasies, I now come home from church and turn on my tape player and hear:

> If someone says, "I love God," and hates his brother, he is a liar; for the one who does not love his brother whom he has seen, cannot love God whom he has not seen. And this commandment we have from Him, that the one who loves God should love his brother also.
>
> 1 John 4:20

Mind-altering, isn't it? Guaranteed to adjust an attitude.

I have invested in a library full of boxed sets of taped messages and Thru the Bible programs, Christian books, and Bible study helps. I deliberately don't spend money on other things so I can make this investment in eternity—not only in my own life but in my family's and the lives of those I touch (and loan my tapes to).

Because of this one practice of listening to Scripture, I absorb God's Word for hours a day. As a wife, mother of five, writer, businesswoman, Bible teacher, and church worker, I would never have the time to spend so many hours in God's Word if I couldn't take it along to listen to while I work. Thank God for modern technology!

With my mind, I participate in deep study of the Word of God. The inductive study method has been especially helpful, since it teaches people to glean from each biblical book what the author wanted to say in context and with proper interpretation. Bible teacher Kay Arthur uses this method, teaching her students to outline the biblical book first, study in context, and do word studies in Hebrew and Greek. This so amplified my understanding of Scripture, and I enjoyed it so much, that I eventually took courses to become a Precept Bible teacher myself.

Through in-depth study, you too can come to know God and his Word in a way you never dreamed possible. And there is still so much to learn! Even in eternity, we'll never get enough of our wonderful Lord, will we? Here and now, we can learn how truth translates into daily life. We can watch how God works—the same powerful way he worked in the lives of Old and New Testament saints. He never changes!

Through this in-depth study, my faith is growing. I have experienced terrible times in life when I've been in a miserable or nightmarish trial. But when I attend my Bible study group—either as a teacher or as a student—I simply float home. My circumstances are the same, but I've been able to rise above them through the revelation and encouragement of spiritual truth.

With my heart, I store God's Word. As I discover valuable verses in my reading, hearing, and studying, I put them to memory. That way I can always have them when they're needed. I highlight verses that jump out at me while reading or studying. Then I write them on three-by-five cards and carry them wherever I go—at home or in the car—to work on those verses until memorized. The list of new verses continues to grow. Sometimes a whole chapter, or even a book, will beg to be put to memory. I've done that too—and reaped the blessing that we receive when we bury the treasure of God's Word in our hearts.

Scripture memorization has at least three key benefits. First, God has a way of bringing back those learned truths just when we need them, for example, when we're tempted to sin or going through a difficult time. The Holy Spirit knows which verse will perfectly strengthen or comfort us at that moment. Like King David, we should pray: "Your word have I treasured in my heart, that I might not sin against You" (Ps. 119:11).

Second, memorization allows us to have a ready word available for witnessing. The Holy Spirit can take what we've put into our hearts and use it to win others to the Lord. Memorize the Roman Road, the Scripture road that leads to salvation in Christ: Romans 3:23; 6:23; 5:8; and 10:9–10. John 3 is also a helpful chapter in leading someone to a saving knowledge of Christ.

Third, memorized truths also come in handy during apologetics—those times when we are called on to defend our faith. Bible teacher Jack Van Impe credits his fruitful ministry with a knowledge of Scripture. Jack has even memorized whole books of the Bible. He puts a disciplined plan into action, which is available on his web site: www.jvim.org.

With my voice, I proclaim the Word through teaching, witnessing, praising, and also training my children. What goes in will come out. This is as true of the positive as the negative. When I go days in a row without spending time in God's Word—reading, hearing, studying, and memorizing—I tend to want to keep my mouth closed. I feel like I don't have anything to say. No word of witness, no defense of the faith, hardly a praise. Like Samson of old, I lose my strength!

If you experience this too at times, the remedy is simple: Get back into the Word. Immerse yourself in it. Overdose on Scripture, and you'll be back to your position of power. God will be able to use you to influence your world.

With my body, I obey the Scripture that God impresses on me. When the Holy Spirit convicts me with truth, I am quick to repent of the sin and bring my life into line with his will. Some sins have taken more time to overcome, like besetting sins—gossiping, lying, unkindness, anger, etc. These are deeply ingrained and are often a part of our personalities.

As my husband and I teach the Bible to our children, we insist that our family live by God's commandments. We can't be hearers (readers, students, etc.) only, but must also be doers of God's Word. Jesus said, "If you love Me, you will keep My commandments" (John 14:15). Our obedience to the Word proves our love for our Savior.

Group Bible study can also help you become obedient. Close fellowship and accountability with other believers is vital to growth as a Christian.

I want you to know that I haven't shared my personal practices to make anyone feel guilty! Instead, I hope to share the incredible difference Bible study has made in my life and to challenge you to commit yourself to scriptural intake. Get excited about all Scripture can do for your life!

Both of us want to add a disclaimer to this section about personal disciplines. We're the first to admit that we're not perfect in this. Busy times go by when we're not able to do all we want to. Other times we get lazy and don't do what we should. But the key thing is that we're consistent. We faithfully take in God's Word every day through some avenue, at some level. This has made the difference in our lives.

As we Christians read, hear, study, memorize, share, and obey God's Word, we'll have the peace and purity that brings light to our eyes. Proverbs 15:30 reads: "Bright eyes gladden the heart." When we have Christ's light and joy in our eyes, others are cheered, encouraged, and attracted to us. Maybe with enlightened eyes like these, we'll be able to use less cosmetic enhancement! For sure, the balance in our lives will be evident to everyone we meet.

6

Loose Lips
or Luscious Lips?

Years ago, four-year-old Carly and I (Cynthia) were in the car on the way to the mall. When a red light stopped us at an intersection, I busied myself searching for something in my purse. Carly, a tiny towhead, pulled down the visor and gazed intently into the mirror. I barely glanced at my daughter as she twisted her face into all sorts of contortions. But she really got my attention when she puckered up and declared, "I've got luscious lips!"

Carly's personal assessment made me laugh that day—how true it is that we females, no matter our age, want luscious lips. Pretty lips. Soft and kissable lips. We know that our eyes and our mouths are the focal points of our faces. Our smiles—accessories more beautiful than flashing jewels—are almost as important as our eyes in expressing our inner selves. If the eyes are the windows of our souls, our mouths are the doors!

Jesus once said, "It is not what enters into the mouth that defiles the man, but what proceeds out of the mouth" (Matt.

15:11). We could paraphrase to say that it's not what we wear on our lips that matters; it's the words of our mouths that must be acceptable.

> Let the words of my mouth and the meditation of my heart
> Be acceptable in Your sight,
> O LORD, my rock and my Redeemer.

Psalm 19:14

In this chapter, we will offer tips to take care of your lips. We'll reveal secrets on lipsticks and liners, cremes, crayons, and lip conditioners. We'll also share thoughts on how our mouths can please both God and people.

Laugh Lines

Generally, our lips are overused and abused. Exposed to the elements and bad habits, our lips reap the chapped, rough skin that develops. As we age, we also accumulate tiny lines around our mouths that are no laughing matter. A few quick care tips will alleviate some of these problems before we add color.

Give Rough Skin the Rub

You learned to exfoliate (remove the top layer of) your facial skin; the same procedure will benefit your lips. Many products on the market can exfoliate for you. Or you can simply rub your lips firmly with a warm washcloth, a facial loofah, or even a toothbrush. Scrub your entire mouth gently, even those horrid lip lines, then rinse with warm water. This will remove the top layer of rough, dead, dry skin and prepare your lips for the next step.

Beautify with Balm

The new, fresh skin is ready for a rich moisturizer. A balm or emollient (rich in oils and lipids) will soften and smooth your lips. You can buy specially prepared lip balms or use something as simple as Vaseline. Just make sure it has a rich texture with lots of oil—it can even feel greasy to touch. Massage it into your lips and surrounding skin. If applied before bed, leave the balm on all night. When applied in the morning before going out, let it sit for ten minutes or so, if you can. Tissue it off just before you put on lip color.

And don't forget your teeth. There's nothing worse than perfectly made-up lips; then the woman smiles and reveals nasty gray or yellow teeth. Many of the foods we eat and drink stain our teeth; also, teeth discolor as we age. We recommend regular home dental care, routine cleanings by a dental hygienist, and if necessary, tooth-lightening products at home or procedures by your dentist. Remember to brush your tongue and use mouthwash for any breath problems. A classy (and kissable) lady always has fresh, clean breath!

Pucker Power

Nothing adjusts a girl's attitude like a new tube of lipstick. That fresh color is often just what you need to perk up tired looks and a weary spirit. Estee Lauder Cosmetics reported that their lipstick index shot way up after the September 11, 2001, terrorist attack on America. The company explained that women buy lipstick (and other cosmetics) when they want an instant pick-me-up but can't afford something bigger.

Women have been loving this glamorous cosmetic for over five thousand years. The product is truly "tested by time"! But lip color has come a long way since women stained their lips with berry juice. Now lipsticks and other products include wax (for smoothness and shine), lipids (for moisturizing), silica (in matte products), UV protection (as sunscreen), even herbs and vitamins, fragrances and flavors, in addition to color.

> In third-century A.D., Talmudic law forbade Jewish women to apply makeup on the Sabbath, but it balanced things out by requiring Jewish husbands to give their wives ten dinars for cosmetics.

Lip colors come in tubes, pots, wands, crayons, and pencils. You can select cremes, glosses, mattes, and frosts in a variety of hues. With lip products, you can match your mood for the day, harmonize with a favorite outfit, or dress up for a special occasion. To decide what works best for you, answer a few questions:

1. Do you feel most in control using a pencil or crayon, a lipstick tube, a lip brush, or a fingertip? Does perfection turn you on? If so, you might like the precision of a pencil or the coverage of a lip brush. Loved finger painting as a kid? Stock up on little pots full of colored gloss. Are you always in a hurry? Nothing beats the simplicity of a quick swipe of lipstick from a tube.
2. What appeals to you—Hollywood starshine or an understated matte finish? Do you want a professional style for business, a natural outdoorsy look, or are you a perpetual glamour girl?
3. Do you enjoy reapplying lipstick every few hours, or would you prefer an all-day color?
4. What color family is best for you—cool or warm? Do you look striking in hospital-white shirts? If so, cool lipsticks will turn you into a knockout. Your

reds, roses, and pinks should have a blue cast to them. Do cream and ivory bring out your complexion better? Then you have warm coloring, and your lipsticks should have yellow or golden undertones.

Mouth Makeovers from a Model

Charity has picked up a few tricks while working with the pros. Here are a few of them.

Lip shades are the only cosmetic you need to coordinate with clothing. They don't have to match exactly, just complement one another. If you're wearing red, you need a red (or a more subtle rose) lipstick. If you're a "cool," it should be blue-red; if a "warm," tomato red. The same goes for your other colors, except blues, greens, etc., which *most* people agree don't look natural on lips. Try contrasts: With a bright or dark blue or black suit, wear red; green looks great with coral or burgundy lips; plum or lavender-pink blend with a purple dress. Have fun experimenting with color!

Any woman can wear red lipstick, but it has to be the right shade of red. And the rest of your face must stay in balance. You don't want to attend a meeting like I (Charity) did, wearing only a big bright mouth! Be sure you have eye-catching brows. Your eyes should be darkened with some mascara and liner, at the very least. Brush on a little blush so your complexion doesn't look washed-out when compared to the intense color of your lips. Red lips can be dynamite when you are going to town for the evening and plan to paint it red.

If red's the last thing you want to see some days, opt for a natural look. Line your lips with a shade closest to your natural lip color, then cover your entire lips with the same. Apply some gloss and you're good to go, a natural beauty who looks better than nature ever intended.

Want just a kiss of color? Line lips with pencil and apply a favorite lipstick. Press lips together for even color, then blot on a tissue. Continue blotting until the color fades. Dot a bit of gloss or frost in the center of each lip. Press together again, spreading the sheen, and presto, you have kissable lips!

Pretty in pink? When magazine editors want models to have that perfect pink pout for the camera, they want more than photogenic facial expressions. Makeup artists work their magic, and you can too! After lining lips with pencil, the artists apply color to both lips. The bottom tint is lighter but from the same color family (any shade will do). In this case, don't press your lips or blot—you'll mix the colors. Finish with a smidgen of gloss in the center of the lower lip.

You need to know the tools of the modeling trade. Most makeup artists use lip brushes to apply color. They feel that the coverage is more complete and that they have more control. Makeup artists mix shades of color frequently. The brush allows them to mix and then blend with ease.

At home, I use lip pencil a lot and love it. It gives a sharper line and a better shape. For better control when you are lining lips, makeup artists suggest holding the lip pencil close to the point.

A full-coverage technique is to apply lip pencil all over your lips. It stays longer than regular creme lipsticks. Then top it off with a frosty gloss or even Vaseline for a quick shine.

If you do decide to wear goopy lipstick, watch that it doesn't end up on your teeth. Do what models do: Say "Ooh" and stick your pointer finger into your mouth. Press your lips against your finger and pull it out. The extra lipstick will come off on your finger.

Want extra-full lips without collagen injections? Line lips with pencil a shade deeper than your lip color. The line can be slightly outside your own natural lip line, if desired. Apply lipstick, then more lip pencil over that. This layering technique is a favorite with makeup artists.

If you aren't crazy about the shape of your mouth, you can create a new one. Cover lips with foundation and powder as a primer. Line lips just above or below your natural lip line, depending on what it is you'd like to change. You can define the bow of your mouth, enlarge your lower lip, curve the corners. Light, frosty colors enlarge; deep, neutral colors minimize wide mouths. Fill in with the color of your choice.

The Tantalizing Two-Step

It only takes two quick steps to create luscious lips that last until your next kiss:

1. With a creamy, sharpened lip pencil or crayon, line your lips. The pencil can match your lip color or be one shade darker. Begin at the center of your upper lip, carefully defining your Cupid's bow. Then, with tiny, connecting strokes, continue the outline down each side of your lips to the corners. On your bottom lip, begin in the center, and again, work to the outside corners. You can blend the line with a stiff little brush, if desired.

2. Apply lip color from a tube or with a brush, beginning in the center of the upper lip and extending out to each side. Blend the color into your lip liner. On the bottom, begin the color at one corner of your mouth and sweep across to the center. Repeat on the other side. Press lips together to spread color evenly. Optional: Top with gloss.

Lip Service

There are qualities about our mouths that are more important than the shade of our lipsticks. Jesus said that what comes out of a woman's mouth defiles her. In his Word, God has provided some rules to regulate the words of our mouths. The first and most important is to confess Jesus Christ as Lord and Savior, according to Romans 10:9. After conversion, our lips can be used to spread the gospel, just as the apostles did. Our mouths were created to glorify God, giving him praise. Finally, our lips need to be used to bless and build up others.

> Let no unwholesome word proceed from your mouth, but only such a word as is good for edification according to the need of the moment, so that it will give grace to those who hear.
>
> Ephesians 4:29

Psalms and Proverbs have so much good advice that there isn't room to record it all. Once, I (Cynthia) made a list of every verse that deals with the mouth. I would read the list over and over, hoping the truth would rub off. Here are a few feminized samples from Proverbs:

She who restrains her words has knowledge (17:27).

A fool's mouth is her ruin,
And her lips are the snare of her soul (18:7).

When there are many words, transgression is unavoidable,
But she who restrains her lips is wise (10:19).

The one who guards her mouth preserves her life;
The one who opens wide her lips comes to ruin (13:3).

Death and life are in the power of the tongue,
And she who loves it will eat its fruit (18:21).

The Power of the Spoken Word

Words are powerful. And when God speaks, things happen.

At Creation, God spoke . . . and the universe was born.

In a storm, Jesus spoke . . . and the angry sea calmed.

At a funeral, Jesus spoke . . . and life revived.

On the cross, Jesus cried, "It is finished!" . . . and our salvation was complete.

Someday, Jesus will shout . . . and we'll meet him in the air.

When you and I speak, powerful things happen too. Our words have the power to heal, build up, or destroy. Judgments that others make about us stick for life. Performer Karen Carpenter plunged into a fatal case of anorexia after overhearing a fan's careless comment about her hips. The authors have experienced the pain of words personally, both in the saying and receiving. Believe us, we apologize every time our words come back to haunt us.

> "Watch your words. Words are powerful. God used the spoken word to create the earth and he will use spoken words to destroy it."
>
> —supermodel Kim Alexis

We want our words to be a blessing to those who hear them. And we're sure you do too. But so often the Enemy trips us up with our own tongue. Following are some red-flag areas to watch in our lives.

Cynthia Shares

A woman I once knew was a good example of the power of the spoken word. When Patty and Paul (not their real names) went out with our social circle, the woman continually criticized her husband. The poor man couldn't do a thing right. It became embarrassing to socialize with them. Friends dropped off. Finally, my husband and I were the only friends left. We tried to tactfully advise the couple to consider marriage counseling. But in anger, Patty and Paul terminated the friendship.

I told my husband, "I'm afraid for their marriage. They have the sweetest kids. What's going to happen to their family?"

It was just a matter of time before Patty and Paul divorced. The couple fell away from the Lord; each moved in with a non-Christian. Not only was the marriage a casualty of Patty's caustic tongue, but so were her lovely children.

As women who seek godliness, we can learn a lot from a mentor God provided in Proverbs 31. This woman was a combination of Martha Stewart, Princess Grace, and Mother Teresa. What Proverbia (as I call her) put her mind to, Proverbia accomplished. Soap operas and talk shows entertained other women; Proverbia stayed busy from morning to night caring for her family and working her business. And the amazing thing is, she did it all with a sweet attitude! Proverbs 31:26 says, "She opens her mouth in wisdom, and the teaching of kindness is on her tongue."

As I raised my young children, I made the two qualities of wisdom and kindness the rule for my tongue. Now that I have teenagers, my resolve has been severely tested. I often have to pray this phrase my kids learned from a movie: "Lord, shut my big yapper!" When I realize that I've spoken hurtful words (or they've been brought to my attention), I ask forgiveness and make it right. We can seek to undo the damage done by using our words to heal.

Swearing

A beautiful woman does not swear or cuss. Period. We might see a gorgeous, classy-looking woman and admire her from afar. Then we get close to her and hear what comes out of her mouth. Jesus is right. Her words defile her! She no longer seems beautiful to us. And yet, in America, we have our loveliest actresses on the screen cussing up a verbal storm. And no one complains about it—we just allow it to continue, setting precedent for us and our children. Foul language is an appalling habit; and that's just what it is, a bad habit.

One of the most pervasive practices is taking the Lord's name in vain. Today even Christians have been heard saying, "Oh my God . . ." They are bombarded with the phrase from television, from movies, on the streets. We can't really judge them. But sadly, their words judge them. Our modern Christian culture takes the third commandment so lightly. Out of reverence, the Jews would not even speak the name of God because his name was so holy. In the Old Testament, it says that the person using the Lord's name in vain should be put to death! That's how strongly God feels about this issue.

Thankfully, we live in the age of grace. But what God hated then, he hates today. Here's a prayer for all of us right now:

Dear Lord, have mercy on us! We are surrounded by people who don't know that you are Creator God. They don't see your beauty or might or wisdom. They don't realize that you loved them enough to die for them. And they treat your name as unholy. Many times a day we hear blasphemous words. They influence us. Please help us impact our culture more than it impacts us. Forgive us for the times we've unwittingly taken your name in vain. Forgive us for the times we disrespected you in order to be cool, to be one of the crowd. Help us to be Christlike in all that we do and say. Let the words of our mouths be pleasing and acceptable to you, O Lord. Amen.

Cynthia Shares

I learned not to gossip the hard way many years ago. At that time in my life, like Robin Hood and his Merry Men, I joined up with a gossipy group. While Robin and his men romped through Sherwood Forest doing good (albeit, stealing from the rich to feed the poor), our band of merry women went around starting forest fires. James 3:5–6 has this to say: "The tongue is a small part of the body, and yet it boasts of great things. See how great a forest is set aflame by such a small fire! And the tongue is a fire, the very world of iniquity; the tongue is set among our members as that which defiles the entire body, and sets on fire the course of our life, and is set on fire by hell."

Strong words for such a little organ—the tongue. Yet our tongues are the very instruments we use to cause great troubles for ourselves and others. In my case, God finally reined in my wayward tongue. This particular group of ladies was good at causing strife. I'm ashamed to admit this time in my life. But if it can help you at all, then I'll share it.

One time, a bit of "news" that I had helped spread got back to the woman. She was very hurt. Phone lines were buzzing all over our small town. With my apology ready, I tried to call until midnight, but her phone was busy. Finally, I recruited my husband to accompany me while I asked forgiveness.

Driving over there, I so desperately wanted to tame my tongue. This wasn't the first time it had gotten me into a heap of trouble. I decided to put James 5:16 into practice: "Confess your sins to one another, and pray for one another so that you may be healed." It only took me one time of doing that to learn to hold my tongue and to stay away from people who don't!

Lying

Our society also takes lying lightly. Most of us have told "little white lies," "stretches of the truth," exaggerations, etc. It's hard to know what the truth is anymore or who you can trust. It's almost expected that certain professions won't tell the truth—salespeople, attorneys, politicians, and so on. Society hardly considers lying a sin these days. But God does.

His Word says that he hates liars. And Revelation 21:8 says that liars won't make it to heaven:

> "But for the cowardly and unbelieving and abominable and murderers and immoral persons and sorcerers and idolaters and *all liars,* their part will be in the lake that burns with fire and brimstone, which is the second death" (emphasis ours).

In that verse, we liars are lumped together with murderers and idolaters, adulterers and abominable folks. God must really hate lying! The sin comes from his enemy. Satan is the father of lies, God says, and there is no truth in him. Revelation 21:8 is most likely talking about unrepentant, unforgiven liars who aren't relying on Christ's sacrifice to save them, who keep practicing their sin, but . . . let's not take any chances! With God's help, let's clean up our act—or mouth, rather. Next time our husbands ask how much we paid for a new dress, let's tell the truth!

Gossip

One of the worst things we can use our mouths for is to criticize and judge others. Gossip and slander are in the list of some of the things God hates.

Are you also sick of your ailing tongue? Misery loves company, right? It might benefit you to hear the story of a spiritual superstar who had the same problem. A favorite Bible heroine, Miriam was blessed with many gifts and talents. One of the most prominent was her gift of gab. Think of how sharp this girl was to answer Pharaoh's daughter in the way that she did, asking if the princess needed a nursemaid for her newfound son and intending to fetch her mother. Miriam was only about twelve years old at the time. She definitely knew how to "think on her feet"—in our day, she would have made a great attorney or politician.

As the women's ministry leader for the Hebrew congregation, this prophetess allowed God to use her tongue for praising him and building up his people. After the miraculous parting of the Red Sea, Miriam composed a song and led the women in singing it. Dancing with tambourines, she sang: "Sing to the LORD, for He is highly exalted; the horse and his rider He has hurled into the sea" (Exod. 15:21).

Though this tune never made the Top 10 hits, the song was probably a favorite chorus back then. Obviously, Miriam was a gifted communicator. But one afternoon (according to Numbers 12), her mouth got her into big trouble.

She and her brother Aaron began slandering Moses. The ringleader of this coup d'état, Miriam said, in so many words, "What was our baby brother thinking when he married that wife of another race? Aaron, you know those Cushites have always been good for nothing. And besides, Moses sets himself above us. Who does he think he is? Don't forget, I used to diaper that boy! If it wasn't for me, he'd still be floating down the Nile. Probably end up crocodile bait! After all, he's not the only one who hears from the Lord. I get a message from God now and then—and I'm not afraid to deliver it. Our little brother's a wimp, Aaron. Why, just the other day . . ."

Suddenly the Lord's voice thundered into the tent. "Moses, Aaron, and Miriam, you three come out to the tent of meeting" (v. 4).

Coming down, enveloped by a cloud, the Lord called Aaron and Miriam to step toward him. Remember the part of *The Wizard of Oz* when the weary travelers—Dorothy, the Scarecrow, the Tin Man, and the Cowardly Lion—are called forward to speak with the great Oz? As they approach the wizard, the foursome cling to each other, knees knocking, teeth chattering. At this point in our Bible story, we chuckle when we imagine Aaron and Miriam coming forward in this same way: hanging on to one another, shaking in their sandals. But unlike the wizard's magic, God's awesome power is real, and the consequence of this sin isn't funny.

The Lord gives the pair quite a lecture. Praising Moses, the Lord asks how they dared to speak against God's servant. Scripture says that the anger of the Lord burned against Moses' sister and brother (v. 9).

Why do we think Miriam instigated this verbal forest fire? For one, her name is mentioned first in the account (and usually women are listed after the men in Scripture). But more importantly, the prophetess receives the punishment. When the cloud of God withdraws, Miriam discovers she is leprous. White as snow, Scripture reports. Leprosy was the most feared plague of that day. The disease results in terrible damage to the flesh of the victim, just as Miriam's words devoured the reputation of her brother. Considered to be very contagious, lepers were always banished from the camp.

And that's just what happened to poor Miriam. She was cast out of the camp.

Moses had mercy on her, however, and cried to the Lord, "O God, heal her, I pray!" (v. 13).

The Lord relented, commanding Miriam to stay outside the camp for seven days. "Afterward she may be received again," he graciously added (v. 14).

Miriam, the girl who loved to talk, spent a whole week by herself. Solitary confinement. No one to chat with. No phone, no Internet. But there was someone with her. And don't you imagine that, with all that time to think, Miriam had quite a few things to say to the Lord, beginning with, "I'm sorry. Forgive me, Lord. Please tame my tongue!"

Thankfully, we live in the age of grace. If not, leprosy might also have been the schoolmaster for many of us. In chapter 3,

James reminds us that we can't curse our brother and praise the Lord too:

> But no one can tame the tongue; it is a restless evil and full of deadly poison. With it we bless our Lord and Father, and with it we curse men, who have been made in the likeness of God; from the same mouth come both blessing and cursing. My brethren, these things ought not to be this way. Does a fountain send out from the same opening both fresh and bitter water? Can a fig tree, my brethren, produce olives, or a vine produce figs? Nor can salt water produce fresh.
>
> verses 8–12

Our words are powerful. Prisoners have been interviewed who shared the sad story of their parents' influence on their lives. Growing up, the phrase criminals heard often repeated by parents was, "You're so bad, someday you're going to end up in prison." The children lived out their parents' expectations. Our words need to build up and edify others—and especially our own families. Proverbs 14:1 says,

> The wise woman builds her house,
> But the foolish tears it down with her own hands [and, we could add, words].

Let's start today to bless our loved ones beyond belief. A recent survey reported that a husband loves his wife and has good feelings about her when she's treating him nicely. (And what's good for the goose is good for the gander, right, ladies?) Our words are one of the ways we express emotion. Think about how many times you praise or say positive things to a new boss or beau. Try this with your family—-your husband, kids, parents, parents-in-law—and see how it spices up your whole life. It will bring a smile to their faces but also give you lovely lips that offer grace and hope to a needy world.

7

Hands That Walk, Feet That Talk

For a minute, forget about appearances. Hands are valuable tools. They assist us in caring for ourselves and others.

Paul Ciniraj has written a wonderful poem that emphasizes the value of certain hands.

It All Depends on Whose Hands It's In

A basketball in my hands is worth about $19.
A basketball in Michael Jordan's hands is worth about $33 million.
It depends on whose hands it's in . . .

A baseball in my hands is worth about $6.
A baseball in Mark McGuire's hands is worth $19 million.
It depends on whose hands it's in . . .

A golf club is useless in my hands.
A golf club in Tiger Woods's hands is four major golf championships.
It depends on whose hands it's in . . .

A rod in my hands will keep away a wild animal.
A rod in Moses' hands will part the mighty sea.
It depends on whose hands it's in . . .

A slingshot in my hands is a toy.
A slingshot in David's hands is a mighty weapon.
It depends on whose hands it's in . . .

Two fish and five loaves in my hands is a couple of fish
    sandwiches.
Two fish and five loaves in Jesus' hands will feed thousands.
It depends on whose hands they're in . . .

Nails in my hands might produce a bird house.
Nails in Christ Jesus' hands will produce salvation for the
    entire world.
It depends on whose hands they're in . . .

As you see now it depends on whose hands it's in.
So put your concerns, worries, fears, hopes, dreams, fami-
    lies and relationships in God's hands.
Because it depends on whose hands they're in.[1]

We agree. A computer at the hands of Danielle Steele is
worth much more than the one we type on. But we still value
our hands. These days, both of us try to take care of our hands
and nails. That wasn't always the case, however. Charity's nails
were short for a reason—a bad habit of biting them that she
now admits to.

Nail Knowledge

Remember the Yellow Pages ad recommending that you
let your fingers do the walking? That's fine, if you have lovely

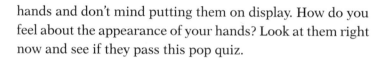

Charity Chats

Yes, admittedly, my hands are one of my most unattractive features. In fact, a friend once told me that she was intimidated when she met me.

"You were like Mary Poppins," she laughs now. "Practically perfect in every way . . . until I saw your hands!"

My hands helped her feel better about herself. So glad I could be of service!

Yes, my hands humble me. If you, too, have a physical feature that humbles you, thank the Lord for it and realize that that very feature can be the thing he uses to glorify himself. We'll talk about the purpose of our hands later in the chapter. For now, let's talk about how to take better care of them.

hands and don't mind putting them on display. How do you feel about the appearance of your hands? Look at them right now and see if they pass this pop quiz.

1. Are my nails uniformly shaped and a practical length for my daily duties?
2. Do my nails look healthy, with no splits and breaks?
3. Do I keep them neatly manicured?
4. Are the knuckles of my hands soft and smooth?
5. What about the skin? Is it as soft and smooth on the palms as the tops of each hand?

If you answered no to any of these questions, we have work to do, and this chapter will give you the information you need to have pleasing hands. Passing the test reveals hands that are in good shape, needing only continued, regular care.

Whose hands are worth special treatment? Yours are! Hands speak volumes to others. They communicate care or

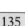

neglect in your grooming. Well-groomed hands and nails show your commitment to every detail of your appearance.

Our friend Terri had this kind of dedication to the condition of her hands. Although she was raising three young sons, her delicate hands never looked like they had washed a dish. Done professionally, Terri's exquisite nails boasted a perfect oval and a polished pink gleam.

Even after she endured two surgeries to remove cancerous brain tumors, suffered through chemotherapy and radiation, lost all her hair, and gained forty pounds from Prednisone, Terri kept up her appointments with the manicurist. We're certain we wouldn't have cared about our hands during a trial like this!

The last time I (Cynthia) saw Terri's hands was in the hospital, the day before Terri died. She had been comatose for several weeks. As she lay there and I prayed for her, Terri's perfect hands were her last vestige of dignity and femininity. I took her weak hand in my own and said to the nurse standing nearby, "Terri has always had the most beautiful hands."

As soon as the words were out of my mouth, Terri's eyes popped open. She looked at me and smiled. Then she went back to sleep. The compliment was my last gift to her.

A Professional Manicure

Do beautiful hands make you, like Terri, feel more respectable and feminine? Want to try your hand at a professional manicure? On the following pages, you'll learn everything you need to know to get salon results. Only this manicure is even better—it's free! Honestly, it takes just minutes each week to maintain properly groomed hands and nails. You can finish off a quick manicure while talking on the phone, watching the news, or visiting with a neighbor. This is the do-it-yourself plan. But it can also be fun to trade manicures with friends, daughters, or sisters.

It helps to start the procedure with everything that you need right at your fingertips. So gather these tools:

Nail polish remover and cotton balls

Emery board

Clippers or scissors

Shallow bowl for soaking cuticles

Nail soak (any mild liquid soap or detergent)

Clean hand towel

Manicure stick or cuticle shaper

Cuticle conditioner

Ridge filler and nail buffer (optional)

Base coat, nail polish, top coat

Hand cream

If you have the necessary materials and some time on your hands, let's begin.

First, as with everything else, start clean and fresh. Remove any old, chipped polish with the remover and cotton balls. Several quick swipes on each nail will do. Trim excess nail with scissors or clippers. You can even do a little bit of shaping this way—not much, so you don't weaken the nail, but this will save time filing. File and shape your nails with an emery board. File toward the center, without sawing back and forth.

Next, fill your bowl with very warm, soapy water. You're going to soak your hands, one at a time, for about a minute each to wash off enamel remover and soften cuticles.

Clean Hands

While our hands are soaking, we can chat. Have you ever noticed others' hands in church? We try not to look around, but sometimes when a lady is raising her hands during worship, we can't help but notice. Especially when they are perfectly manicured with a flashing new color. We admire hands like this; but you know, we don't think attractiveness is what God is looking for. He's seeking the hands that represent a heart submitted to him, hands that are responding to his love and lordship.

The appearance of our hands doesn't matter much to God. Manicured hands are more of a cultural thing. What does matter to God? Clean hands, and I'm not talking about the cleansing that comes from a good soak, like we're doing. Psalm 24:3–4 defines these hands:

Who may ascend into the hill of the LORD?
And who may stand in His holy place?
He who has clean hands and a pure heart.

David continued this thought in another psalm when he said, "I shall wash my hands in innocence" (Ps. 26:6). Hands that please God are clean, not involved with sin. They symbolize a heart that is innocent, pure, and unsoiled. A heart that has repented, sought the Lord's forgiveness, and is wholly following after him.

As we meet with different churches, members come to us with burdens. The hands (and hearts) of many Christians are no longer clean. The story about the minister's wife who ran off with a parishioner has been repeated in various congregations. And pastors are leaving their wives for other women. A worship minister announced to his congregation that he was involved in a homosexual affair. Some youth pastors engage in sex with their young female charges. One such leader recently landed in prison. A pastor's son was permanently expelled from school for illegal activity. Drug and alcohol abuse, bribery and extortion, insurance fraud, violence, pornography, and immorality infect our land—and our churches. A recent survey reveals that the divorce rate is higher in the church than out.

Our hearts are so grieved as we hear these stories. And yet, there was another time and place in history that revealed a sin-sick society like we see today—the days of Noah. How bad was it? Genesis 6:5–6 are probably two of the saddest verses in the Bible:

> Then the LORD saw that the wickedness of man was great on the earth, and that every intent of the thoughts of his heart was only evil continually. And the LORD was sorry that He had made man on the earth, and He was grieved in His heart.

The next chapter of Genesis records God's plan to "blot out man whom I have created from the face of the land . . . for I am sorry that I have made them" (6:7) and to start fresh with Noah and his family.

What a heartbreaking scene!

It's as if a mother would say to one of her children, "I'm sorry I ever gave birth to you!"

But this is God's response to iniquity. He can't tolerate sin. The degree of his own holiness won't allow him to. The Bible tells us that God is merciful, patient, and long-suffering with humanity, waiting for us to repent. But his righteousness does demand justice. He must judge.

As we hear these stories of sin in God's sanctuaries, we know he will judge. We believers are his children. He loves us too much to let us continue in unrighteousness.

Dr. J. Vernon McGee, the beloved radio minister, once said, "If you get by with sin, you're not God's child. The Father only paddles his own children." God chastises us for sin for our own eternal good. Humanly speaking, if a mother loves her children, she will not allow them to continue in bad behavior. When she sees areas of sin in her kids' lives, she will discipline them, no matter how tired, sick, or preoccupied she is. The mother does it for their own good, the good of the family, the good of society, and most importantly, for eternity.

I (Cynthia) have told my children, "We need to be living lives that please the Lord, with no compromise. His commandments must be obeyed down to the punctuation marks. We need clean hands and pure hearts. God is going to judge, and we want to be found righteous."

Revival Starts with One

Despite a world full of sin, God always finds an obedient remnant, even if it dwindles down to just one person.

Genesis 6 also tells us about one man, Noah, who found grace and favor in the eyes of the Lord. He was a righteous man, blameless in his time, a man who walked with God. Noah pleased the Lord, and God saved him out of destructive judgment.

We want to be in that number, don't you?

But how do we ensure that our hands are clean, our hearts pure? If you take Jesus' advice in Matthew 18:8, you'll cut your sinning hand off and throw it away! He told the disciples,

"If your hand or your foot causes you to stumble, cut it off and throw it from you; it is better for you to enter life crippled or lame, than to have two hands or two feet and be cast into the eternal fire."

Ouch! That's tough! We really don't think Jesus wants us to go around maiming ourselves. He's using hyperbole, or exaggeration, in this instance to emphasize the seriousness of sin.

A childhood song reminds us:

> O be careful little hands what you do,
> be careful little hands what you do,
> for the Father up above looks down in tender love,
> be careful little hands what you do.

I (Cynthia) am thankful that my mother slapped my little hand when I reached out to do wrong. We should make this our continual prayer: "Heavenly Father, slap my hand when I reach out to grab sin!"

Clean hands are guaranteed when we continually meditate on the nail-scarred hands of our Savior. Picture Jesus standing before us in compassion, his outstretched arms displaying nail prints caused by the world's sin. Those scars will be reminders for all eternity that the gap between God's holiness and our sinfulness was bridged by the cross.

The disciple Thomas doubted Christ's resurrection. After Jesus was raised, he stood before Thomas with his hands displayed and said, "Reach here with your finger, and see My hands . . . do not be unbelieving, but believing" (John 20:27).

Believe that Jesus lives today to change lives, to give fresh starts, to clean up dirty hands and hearts. Believe! Out of love, Jesus died for our unrighteousness, taking our sins on his own body. Our hands and hearts are washed spotless in the blood of the Lamb.

More Powerful than Borax

Richard Wheeler, an evangelist and friend, visited a butcher shop one day. The butcher's hands were stained and he wanted to clean them up fast.

"I've got some lamb's blood here," he told Richard. "I'll scrub them with that."

Richard thought this was a strange and barbaric practice. But the butcher revealed an interesting fact.

"Sheep's blood has cleansing properties in it," he explained. "If you want to get something clean and white, use sheep's blood."

He proceeded to scour his hands with the lamb's blood, and in a minute, they were spotless.

What a beautiful picture of Christ's sacrifice—the Lamb of God who takes away the sins of the world! "What can wash away my sin?" the song asks. "Nothing but the blood of Jesus," comes the declaration. If you want to get your hands and hearts sparkling clean, repent of the sinful works of your hands and cleanse them from sin (James 4:8) through receiving Jesus' righteousness as your own. The Bible promises a reward:

> The LORD has rewarded me according to my righteousness;
> According to the cleanness of my hands He has recompensed
>   me.
> For I have kept the ways of the LORD,
> And have not wickedly departed from my God.
>
> Psalm 18:20–21

Some day Christians will stand before the judgment seat of Christ and be rewarded for the works of their hands here on earth. We had better get busy, hadn't we?

The Prescription for Sin

If our hands have sinned, all we need to do is simply confess it. We can't hide anything from God anyway. He even knows our thoughts. The poet John Greenleaf Whittier once wrote, "Our thoughts lie open to Thy sight, and naked to Thy glance. Our secret sins are in the light of Thy pure countenance." Our lives are an open book in God's kingdom. Dr. Lewis Sperry Chafer, founder of Dallas Theological Seminary, has said, "Secret sin down here is open scandal in Heaven."

The wisest thing to do is to confess sin as soon as it happens. This ensures unbroken fellowship between the Lord and us. The story is told about the great nineteenth-century preacher Charles Spurgeon, who was walking with a friend. As Spurgeon crossed a busy street, suddenly he stopped in the middle with bowed head. To his friend, already waiting on the other side of the street, it looked like Charles was praying. When Charles had finally crossed, the friend demanded, "What were you doing out there? You could have been run over by a carriage!"

"Praying," Spurgeon answered matter-of-factly.

"What was so important that it couldn't wait until you crossed the street?" The friend was perplexed.

"A cloud came between me and my Savior," Spurgeon replied. "I wanted to remove it before I got to the other side of the street."

Spurgeon knew. Unbroken fellowship with God is worth risking life and limb. Our Lord desires clean hands and hearts. We must do whatever it takes to keep them that way.

Back to Beauty

At this stage in our manicure, we're ready to dry off our hands and push back our cuticles. You can use the blunt, rounded end of a manicure stick. Or you know what else works great? A pencil eraser! The soft cushion of a clean pencil eraser gives just the right pressure without scratching. You want to push back your cuticles regularly (say daily, after dishes or a bath) to train them. The lunule of the nail (or the half-moon at the base) should be visible. This adds length to the nail bed and creates a pleasing effect. Apply cuticle conditioner to cuticles that need more softening.

If your nails call for it, you can apply ridge filler and/or buff your nails. Always buff at an angle in one direction.

If your hands tend to be rough and dry, a secret pampering treatment might be just what the manicurist ordered. Massage some emollient into your hands. Work it in well. Then, leaving the emollient on, take an exfoliant scrub. (You can buy it at any drugstore. It will have some sort of grainy properties, like crushed almonds or oatmeal, to rub off the top layer of skin.) Rub the scrub all over your hands, especially working on rough areas like knuckles and wrists. Then, without removing the emollient or scrub, squirt several drops of a creamy wash or dish detergent into your palms. Wash your hands with the lather and rinse well. You can actually feel the rough, dry skin going down the drain! Don't your hands feel satiny smooth now?

Dry with your towel, and get ready for some fun. Choose enamel in a favorite shade or in a color to match your outfit for a special event. Make sure nails are free of any oil. If you want, you can brush on a base coat and let it dry. Base and top coats help your manicure last longer. Apply polish with three quick strokes—one down the middle of the nail and one on each side. Begin with the pointer finger of each hand, working through the fingers to the pinky, leaving the thumb last. Otherwise, if you polish the thumb first, you may smudge it when you tip your hand to get to your other fingers. You can apply several coats, if you want, allowing time to dry between each application. Complete with a top coat, brushing it under the tips of your nails for added protection. Again, allow to dry.

For a soft, smooth finish, massage in hand cream, concentrating on rough knuckles. Lotion with sunscreen prevents brown spots.

A professional manicure should last about one to two weeks, depending on how often you have your hands in water and solutions. We have some methods, however, that can preserve your efforts. First, use latex gloves when you do dishes or heavy scrubbing. Second, use gloves in the garden, which safeguards your hands against sun and soil damage and protects your manicure.

In our next book, *The Healthy Balance*, we share nutritional tips to nourish you from head to toe, inside and out. This includes having healthy nails too, and we have some advice that may help your nails grow:

- Bone up on calcium. This mineral is not only good for your bones and teeth but your nails as well. Make sure you are getting 1,000 mg daily from dairy products, greens, nuts, tofu, and/or supplements.
- Buy some biotin. This vitamin, also known as B-7, helps your nail-cell growth. Thirty to 100 mcg daily is what you need.
- Load up on B-12 bombers. Also in the B vitamin family, B-12, or cobalamin, aids in nail-cell formation and absorption of protein. You can get your B vitamins from brewer's yeast, dairy products, eggs, sea vegetables, broccoli, whole grains, or supplements.
- Bring blood flow to your cuticles and nail bed with a massage. Warm olive oil and massage it into your cuticles

Cynthia Shares

Unlike my daughter Carly, who was born with beautiful hands, my motley mitts were never particularly attractive. They bothered me until I read this statement:

*The beauty of the hands is not in their appearance
but in what they can do.*

I was relieved to know this, since my hands actually can do quite a lot. I take good care of my husband and children, which is God's will according to Titus 2:3–5. I play the piano for worship and teach a pack of piano students. My hands make meals, pies, cakes, and other goodies for the sick and elderly. My hands aid my Bible teaching. I help ladies look and feel good. My writing and publishing has spread the gospel message around the world.

I've noticed that Charity communicates with her hands—as she speaks, as she sings, as she praises God. The way she expresses God's transforming love through her hands is truly beautiful. In both Charity's life and mine, our hands have sometimes become the hands of Christ as we have touched others with the Lord's healing caress.

and clean nails. Leave on one hour, then wash off and rub in hand cream.

Desirable Hands

After a good manicure, your hands are a desirable feature to be proud of. Do you know the type of hands God desires? Holy hands (1 Tim. 2:8). Hands set apart for him. Now that your hands look so nice, be sure that you use them in service for the Lord.

Answer these questions in your "New You" Notebook: What can your hands do for the Lord? Do you have a talent or a skill to offer? Could you create something to share with the body of Christ? There is no limit to what the Holy Spirit will do with hands that are open to him in submission.

A First-Century Fashion Designer

A New Testament lady named Dorcas used her hands for the Lord. She was a seamstress whose creative gifts provided clothing for the needy in the early church. Acts 9:36 says that she "was abounding with deeds of kindness and charity which she continually did." Dorcas's beautiful hands were so loved and needed by the people that when she grew ill and died, they sent for Peter to come revive her. In the midst of the tears, Dorcas's friends showed Peter all the tunics and garments she had made them.

The story has a happy ending. The power of the Holy Spirit raised Dorcas, who went on to create many more high fashions of the first century. God gave us hands for a reason: More than just to look pretty, they can reach out to a hurting world with the love of Jesus Christ.

Feet for Walking

Our feet also have a special calling. Like our hands, they too can be beautiful. We don't need to spend much time on these extremities. Usually they are covered with shoes, thank goodness! But it's important to wear stylish but comfortable shoes. Find a nice balance between comfort and style.

PediCare

Your feet are probably the most abused part of your body. You walk on them, stub your toes every so often, squeeze them

Cynthia Shares

Some of us occasionally choose comfort over style, as was the case at a speaking engagement that I had several years ago. I was scheduled to speak at a large Christian event in a neighboring city. In a house full of five kids, it's always an adventure getting ready to attend anything. But when I go to speak, not only do I have to "dress to impress," I have to gather up all my books for my book table and make sure I get out the door on time with book boxes, purse, Bible, and hopefully my notes for my talk.

This day I was quite proud of myself when I arrived early at the church with all of the above and was escorted down to the front of the auditorium. I greeted people and chatted happily, oblivious to a glaring defect. When my name was announced and the introduction began, I glanced around the huge sanctuary. A few butterflies quivered in my stomach as I observed thousands of people in attendance. Then my stomach hit the floor when I looked down at my feet. I was wearing my bedroom slippers! And not just any bedroom slippers—these were furry monsters I had been given at Christmas! They had been so comfortable that I had run out of the house in them. The only choice I had, other than making a worse fool of myself by bawling loudly as I ran down the aisle and out the back door, was to march onstage and tell a funny story at my own expense. Take it from one who knows—a nice balance between comfort and style works best!

into tight shoes, and stand on them for what seems an eternity. But a little attention helps our feet look and feel better.

For a quick pedicure, collect these materials:

Enamel remover and cotton balls

Clippers

Manicure stick

Nail brush

Emery board

Pumice stone

Tub and detergent for soaking

Dry towel

Moisturizer

Nail enamel

To begin, use the nail clipper to cut each toenail straight across, following the shape of your toe. Don't allow toenails to grow longer than the end of your toe.

Smooth jagged edges with the emery board, working toward the center in one direction.

Remove old polish before soaking your feet in a large basin (or the tub) filled with very warm, soapy water for about ten minutes (this is the relaxing part, so if you have more time, enjoy!). During this soak, you can use the pumice stone to soften rough skin and calluses. Scrub your toenails with the nail brush to rid them of dirt and grime. Or like us, forget it all and read a book! Towel dry your feet.

Push back the cuticles with the manicure stick and apply polish, if desired.

Finish with a nice massage (given by you or a loved one—if your feet aren't ticklish), working the moisturizer into your skin.

Feet That Talk

Giving yourself a pedicure every so often feels great. And it shows our feet the respect they deserve for serving us so faithfully. In biblical times, care for feet came in the form of a foot-washing. Traveling those dusty Roman roads in sandaled feet required some personal attention at the end of the day. Usually it was the servants who did the pedicures, or foot-washings, in Bible times. But the Bible tells of several special occasions where foot-washing symbolized so much more than outward cleanliness.

Two New Testament women demonstrated their love for the Savior by cherishing his feet. One lady washed Jesus' feet with her tears, afterward drying them with her long hair. Another follower of Christ used costly perfume (worth a year's wages) to anoint his feet. Jesus was so pleased with her act of love that he promised it would be remembered forever.

> "Love is not theory or talk, but deeds. It is doing what needs to be done in every situation."
>
> —source unknown

Jesus cared for his disciples' feet when he humbly knelt at the last Passover supper, washing them as a servant would. Christ did this as an example to them and to us. Jesus' humility provides a reminder to serve him by serving others.

The late Roman Catholic Bishop Fulton J. Sheen once stated, "Show me your hands. Do they have scars from giving? Show me your feet. Are they wounded in service? Show me your heart. Have you left a place for divine love?"[2]

God created our feet, and he thinks they are lovely, but not just in appearance. "How beautiful are the feet of those who preach the gospel," Romans 10:15 says. Have your feet taken you somewhere to share Christ? Then they are beautiful!

We know two wealthy ladies who moved to gorgeous Baja Beach, below Ensenada, Mexico, to retire. Phyllis and June lived in luxury on the edge of the Pacific, drove shiny new Cadillacs, and had everything they needed and desired. Their plan was to relax and enjoy life in their "golden years."

But one day, their feet took them into one of the Oaxacan (Waw-haw-kun) Indian camps. The Oaxacans come up to Baja from the most southern state in Mexico looking for work. They are some of the poorest people on the face of the earth.

These two ladies saw the poverty: children with no clothes and shoes, some of them running around the camp naked; one twelve-year-old boy wore a flowered dress because that was all he owned. Many children hadn't eaten in days. There was sickness, filth. Homes were made out of cardboard, mattresses, plastic—anything they could find in the garbage. Whole families existed in these tiny dwellings, from grandma and grandpa down to the newest member. One woman lived in a one-room shanty with her eleven young children. Sewage ran past the hut on the dirt path, and a toddler played in it.

Phyllis and June witnessed all of this, but they also saw the spiritual poverty. They began visiting the camps once a week, bringing Phyllis' accordion to play gospel choruses and an interpreter to translate Bible stories. At the end of the story time, shared with eight children under an olive tree, the ladies passed out fruit. But when they returned the following week, the newly enlisted missionaries taught the Bible to over seventy people.

"Of course, they may have been coming for the bananas," June laughs. "But at least they heard the gospel!"

That was in 1987. Today there is a mission complex at the site called Helping Hands, complete with a Christian school, a church with several services a week, medical facilities where doctors volunteer their time, a distribution program for clothes and food, and much more. The good news that Christ saves is going out to hundreds on a daily basis. All because two "retired" ladies were willing to let their feet take the gospel wherever it was needed.

Evangelist Billy Graham was once quoted in the *Chicago American*, saying, "The most eloquent prayer is the prayer through hands that heal and bless. The highest form of worship is the worship of unselfish Christian service. The greatest form of praise is the sound of consecrated feet seeking out the lost and helpless."

Are we willing to step out in faith and follow Jesus, no matter where he leads—to our neighbor's door or even across the sea in the name of Christ? Our hands and feet can be truly beautiful when we use them in God's power to impact our world for eternity.

8

Fragrance of Beauty for Body and Soul

As we move from the top of our heads down to our toes in this transformation journey, one of the most important considerations is cleanliness. We want to smell fresh and clean, whether or not we add any additional fragrances. This is a must for every day, but it is especially important on memorable occasions. Suppose that on your wedding day you decided to do a little gardening. Digging around in the muddy flower bed with the sun shining brightly, you worked up a sweat. When it came time for your wedding ceremony, you wouldn't just step into your gorgeous white gown and ride off into the sunset with Prince Charming, would you? Of course not! Hopefully, the number-one item on your to-do list would be a shower!

Become a Clean Freak

Shining hair, spotless skin, and a fresh, clean body are essential for the beautiful bride, woman, or any person who desires a makeover. When a homeless alcoholic reforms, one of the first thing he or she (or those helping that person) insists on is getting cleaned up. What a difference a bath can make! A bath or shower need not be drudgery. Instead, it can become a favorite part of your day. If you're a shower person, stock up on some sweet-smelling shower gels and loofah brushes for an invigorating scrub. Fragrant lotions finish off your grooming. Or the bathing beauties among us can really turn getting clean into a healthy ritual: a tub full of warm, scented water, a vinyl pillow, soft music, and candlelight will lower your blood pressure while the bubbles lift away the day's grime. Slip into some warm pajamas or a silky gown, and you're ready for bed.

Cleanliness isn't the only reason for taking long, hot baths. We love a good soak when we need to relax. Try putting a few drops of essential oils in your bath water. Mmm, you'll smell great afterwards. You can create your own bath salts by mixing essential oils (from health food stores) with the bath salts. Scents like ylang-ylang, eucalyptus, lavender, rose, sandalwood, and patchouli can relax and rejuvenate you. Create your own recipes, and write them down in your "New You" Notebook.

In a similar fashion, to be spiritually beautiful we must start out fresh and clean. The Bible tells us that our hearts are dirtied by sin. We need a spiritual bath. According to 1 John 1:7, the only thing that can cleanse us from all sin is the blood of Jesus, God's Son. Our heavenly Father loved us so much that, even in our sinful state, he sent his Son to pay the price for our sin. Jesus Christ died on the cross and was buried. But he rose again and lives today to forgive us from sin, filling our hearts with his love and saving grace.

As we travel through life, we'll continue to get dirty. But 1 John 1:9 assures us that "if we confess our sins, He is faithful and righteous to forgive us our sins and to cleanse us from all unrighteousness."

Making Sense of Scents

Now we're ready to add some fragrance to our lives. If you love perfume, you're not alone. Sales from American perfume companies make record profits. However, our human obsession with scent didn't just start in this country or in this century. The use of fragrance goes back at least six thousand years. In ancient times, pagan priests offered perfumes to their gods. Eventually, people learned to employ perfume as healing substances. Fragrant oils were used in trading and given as gifts. Two of the offerings that the Magi brought the Christ child were fragrances: frankincense and myrrh.

Since the eighteenth century, the European town of Grasse, with its warm climate in southern France, has been a primary source of the flowers used to create society's most coveted perfumes. In the 1800s, Paris became the fashion capital of the world. At that time, prestigious perfumeries were established, and French perfumes became famous. Since then, the love of and demand for fine fragrances has traveled around the globe.

It's fun to visit the department stores here in the States to test and experiment with new scents. Your favorites need not be expensive or even popular name brands. But they do have to blend well with your body chemistry. Fragrances smell different on each person.

What aromas appeal to you? Something sweet and floral? A fresh, green, natural scent? Or maybe a perfume that's heavy with oriental notes? Women choose fragrances based on their emotions. Ask yourself: How do I feel when I wear this scent?

Does this smell remind me of someone or something or a special time and place? What does the aroma say about me?

Perfumes are categorized into five general classifications:

- *Florals* contain an essential oil from one specific flower or a combination of flowers known as a floral bouquet. Within this group, scents can range from intensely floral, to softly sweet, or simply fresh. Florals express a romantic personality, very feminine and soft. Some popular perfumes in this category are T Girl by Tommy Hilfiger (a fresh scent), Happy by Clinique, Jessica McClintock (a crisp scent), Romance by Ralph Lauren, Joy by Jean Patou (a classical), Tiffany (a rich scent), and Eternity by Calvin Klein (a crisp, green floral).

- *Fresh and Green* scents are for the fresh, outdoorsy girl. They are alive with the natural aromas of herbs, leaves, ferns, and grasses. One fragrance company even sells a perfume that smells like celery! The aroma of herbs is often blended with the oils of flowers, like carnations or lilies of the valley, adding a subtle sweetness. Favorites in this category are Polo Sport by Ralph Lauren, DKNY by Donna Karan, and Cristalle by Chanel.

- *Orientals,* as exotic as they sound, are composed of ingredients like incense, spices, earthy scents, and vanilla. They make a scented statement that lingers longer than any other fragrance. Orientals are sensual, mysterious, and bold—just like the woman who wears them. Best-selling fragrances in this category are Shalimar by Guerlain, Opium by Yves Saint Laurent, and Magie Noire by Lancôme.

- *Woody Orientals* contain rich oriental notes blended with powerful wood scents like patchouli, sandalwood, and musk. If you love this category, scents to try are Fendi (rich, rich), Angel by Thierry Mugler (green and fruitier),

Charity Chats

My husband, Kel, has a strong sense of smell. When he holds me close (and as newlyweds, we practice that one a lot!), he always whispers, "Mmm, I love the way you smell."

When I ask what he loves about my "personal scent," Kel always replies, "You smell like 'home' to me."

At first, I thought, "That's a weird answer." I mean, who's ever heard of a sexy Liz Claiborne perfume called "Home"? Who'd buy that? Companies choose compelling names for their fragrances like "Obsession" and "Love Spell" for a reason. Women want to drive their men wild, not smell like "home."

For a minute, I felt I'd failed as a female, but then I understood what he meant. My husband was giving me the best compliment: I smelled like home because my "personal scent" is a comfort to him. When Kel smells it, he knows he is near me, finally home, right where he belongs. Each home has its own personal scent, for better or worse. But when you've been gone a long time, aren't you happy to get home where you belong? Let's see if we can find you a fragrance that will make someone special long to come home to you!

Paloma Picasso (a classical chypres), Red by Giorgio (fruitier), Samsara by Guerlain, and Donna Karan (both classical).

- *Water* is a new category. Today's scents are light, clean, and more transparent. These fragrances include marine notes and a scent of sea air. Selections in the category are L'eau D'Issey by Issey Miyake, New West for Her by Aramis, and Escape by Calvin Klein.

Fragrance is created in three layers. The top note is the scent you smell first. What do you smell when you first apply the perfume? The middle layer develops after a few minutes on

Cynthia Shares

I don't have a signature scent because I enjoy many perfumes and wear them according to my mood. I'll ask myself, "What kind of day is it? Do I feel like a natural woman, a spice girl, or a business type today?" I'll wear the scent that best reflects my answer. When I'm going on a picnic or running errands, I spritz on a fresh, natural cologne or use fruit-scented body lotion. At a business meeting or speaking engagement, I make a professional statement with a bold, elegant, long-lasting perfume. A night out on the town with my husband calls for something spicy and sultry. I can predict exactly what he'll like, and I spray it all over my body.

When I dress for church, however, I lighten up on fragrance. I don't want to flare people's allergies during the service and hinder their worship. From my own experience with allergic reactions, I know that a woman's powerful perfume can make sitting in the same room miserable, and sometimes even intolerable. Ann Landers, in one of her columns, suggested wearing fragrance so lightly that it was barely noticeable. "A lovely plus," she called it.

your pulse points. This is the heart of the scent. The third layer comes after the "dry down," when the alcohol in the perfume has evaporated. These are the holding layers containing the oils. In this layer, the perfume notes linger and mellow out. That's why just spraying a scent into the air and sniffing will not give you a good representation of the perfume. It must be worn—the oils in the fragrance mix with your own personal body chemistry and are then released by the warmth of your body.

Your Signature Scent

Some women want to discover their "signature scent." This perfume will express who they are and become a statement of their feminine qualities. To select a signature scent, Barbara Palermo, fragrance consultant with Macy's department stores, suggests that you ask yourself some questions. What natural aromas appeal to you? Which of these outdoor smells do you appreciate—grass, flowers, pine and woods, the ocean? This will help you decide on a fragrance category. The grass-lovers might like Green scents. Do you adore flowers? Of course, choose a Floral. If breathing pine-scented air while standing in a forest appeals to you, the Wood scents are what you want. Love to inhale ocean mist instead? Choose a fragrance from the new Water category.

Now answer these questions: What perfumes have attracted you in the past? Select a scent in the same family. Is there a fragrance that gives you a rush? That's the one for you!

After answering the questions to decide your favorite fragrance category, take this book to a department store fragrance counter. Ask for cards to try some of the perfumes listed. Take the sprayed cards with you while you shop and continue smelling them for awhile. See which fragrances you like and don't like. Then try your two top favorites on each wrist. Wear them around the mall for ten minutes. Which one appeals to you most now? You have found your signature scent. (Over time, if your message about yourself changes, don't be afraid to choose a second signature scent.)

Your special scent represents who you are. You've chosen carefully, ensuring that the blend of fragrances best expresses your unique identity. This perfume can be worn continually and layered with bath and body care products until finally the aroma is identified as your own.

A Memorable Fragrance

So, ladies, let's aim for a "lovely plus" with our perfume application. Choose your fragrance according to the day (or the type of day you'd like to have). And wear it gently.

How did Mary choose the fragrance with which to anoint Jesus' feet? What kind of day was it? Obviously, a day to honor her Savior. And only a pound of pure nard would do. Spikenard, as it is called, was the most precious and priceless of ancient aromatics. Mary's demonstration of worship cost a year's wages, quite a sacrifice. After pouring the perfume on Jesus' feet, then wiping them with her hair, the house filled with the fragrance of the spikenard.

But Judas complained about it. He wasn't concerned with allergies—he decried the expense. Jesus defended Mary's act, however, stating that she had prepared his body for burial. She would always be remembered for this sacrifice, Jesus said. Surely, Mary floated home that day. And think of it. Like Jesus, Mary had been drenched in perfume from the top of her head to her toes. He was reminded of her. And for days afterward, she wore the scent of her Savior (John 12:3–8).

In the same way today, we are to be drenched with the fragrance of Jesus. Our spiritual scent should fill every house that we enter, and those inside should ask, "What is that delightful aroma?"

Have you ever been out in a public place when a stranger walked by wearing the most delicious fragrance? You just had to ask, right? While walking down a city sidewalk one day, I (Cynthia) passed a woman who smelled fantastic. I quickly turned and asked the woman, "Excuse me. Your perfume is wonderful. What is it?"

"Eternity," she replied.

I immediately bought a bottle. In doing so, I acquired a great spiritual object lesson. When we pass by people in our daily lives, the scent of the Savior should be so strong that it stops them in their tracks.

"What's that fragrance?" they'll want to know.

"It's my Savior!" comes our answer. And then we can offer them the hope of the gospel. "Eternity," we'll reply. "Eternity with Christ."

The apostle Paul said it this way in 2 Corinthians 2:14–16:

> But thanks be to God, who always leads us in triumph in Christ, and manifests through us the sweet aroma of the knowledge of Him in every place. For we are a fragrance of Christ to God among those who are being saved and among those who are perishing; to the one an aroma from death to death, to the other an aroma from life to life.

How to Smell Good Spiritually

Ephesians 5:1–2 tells us how we can smell appealing spiritually:

> Therefore be imitators of God, as beloved children; and walk in love, just as Christ also loved you and gave Himself up for us, an offering and a sacrifice to God as a fragrant aroma.

Our love for others is the fragrance that attracts, much like honey-scented blossoms draw bees. It's the sweet aroma of Christ's pure, unconditional compassion. Now we can allow that same love to flow through us to others. Offer those you meet his acceptance, kindness, and grace, expressed through

> "Love is a great beautifier."
>
> —Louisa May Alcott, author of *Little Women*

empathetic eyes and a sincere smile. When people fail us, as we so often do to one another, forgive and restore them to fellowship. We must be gracious and well mannered, treating others as more important than ourselves.

Cynthia Shares

My paternal grandmother, Garnette Culp, had a signature scent: Galore. She wore Galore day and night, whether attending a special event, grocery shopping, or just sitting around the house alone, or going to bed. Over time, it seemed that the rich perfume seeped into Grama's pores, and it identified her even more than her sky-blue eyes and musical laugh. When the family smelled Galore, we thought of Grama. This particular aroma exuded from everything Grama touched and from everything that touched Grama: her sheets and towels, couch and chair, her clothes. When coming up the walkway to her house, the special scent greeted us before we reached her door. After our visit, which always included Grama's hugs, we wore the fragrance home.

Several years ago, Grama died and went to heaven, taking her signature scent with her. The day before her funeral, I picked through some of her personal items that had been donated to a church rummage sale. I missed Grama terribly and had asked the Lord for one special keepsake to remember her by. In my search, I noticed Grama's bathroom trash can with something at the bottom. Reaching down, I pulled up the most priceless gift: a small, nearly empty bottle of perfume. I twisted off the cap and breathed deeply of the rich aroma. Mmm, Galore!

Memories of Grama swirled through my head. I still keep that tiny bottle in my dresser drawer. Even though Grama is now in heaven, her memory will always be with me. Her love never leaves me. Every time I want a reminder of Grama, I sniff her signature scent.

Our words should be wise, kind, and edifying. Our touch, full of gentle healing. An aroma to the saved "from life to life," Scripture says.

How can we consistently show God's love to our brothers and sisters in Christ? By dying to our selfishness and self-centeredness. As we surrender our own will and way to conform to the image of Jesus Christ, we become like him. And he is pure love.

Fellow believers will not be the only people to benefit from our Christlike benevolence. Non-Christians will be drawn to the Savior by this unusual demonstration of love. A poem (author unknown) illustrates the responsibility of our witness:

> You are the only Bible some people will read.
> You're writing the gospel, a chapter a day
> by the words that you say,
> and the deeds that you do.
> Men read what you write whether faithless or true;
> say, what is the gospel, according to you?

Your Spiritual Signature Scent

Just like having a signature perfume scent, God wants us to have a spiritual signature scent. What are you known for? Are you a woman of prayer and faith? Do friends appreciate your kindness? Is your life characterized by joy? Do others talk about your physical loveliness or your love? We've noticed that the things others remember us for aren't our looks but our words and actions. They also don't forget the kindnesses and good deeds we've done for them. Christ's love in us is the keepsake that others will always cherish.

Incense before the Throne

We can also be a sweet fragrance unto the Lord. Our godly lives are one of the ways we please him, like a sweet sacrifice. Our prayers are another. Revelation 8:3–4 gives us a new perspective for our prayer life. The scene is heaven, with seven angels standing around the throne of God:

Cynthia Shares

I start my day at the throne of grace—on my knees. I know that I can't make it one moment without God and his help. I need the fullness of the Holy Spirit in my life, and I plead for his power in my children's lives. I pray "without ceasing" throughout the day, but I also include a concentrated prayer time when I bring needs of my own and others to him. Prayer walking (discussed in *The Healthy Balance*) is one way that I regularly exercise my faith while shaping up my body. An occasional prayer ceremony is the other way.

And another angel came and stood at the altar, holding a golden censer; and much incense was given to him, so that he might add it to the prayers of all the saints on the golden altar which was before the throne. And the smoke of the incense, with the prayers of the saints, went up before God out of the angel's hand.

When we pray, our prayers go up before God's throne. Prayer releases supernatural power, providing for the physical and spiritual needs of us and our loved ones. But even more important, our prayers are a form of worship. They rise up to God like savory incense. Our prayers surround him with the passion of our hearts and the submission of our souls.

When you pray, take time to sit and bask in God's presence. Don't say a word—just worship. Close your eyes. Shut out any distractions. Allow the emotion to well up from deep within. Offer your worship to the Almighty, just as Mary offered her perfume. Raise your hands to him, open-palmed, relinquishing the rule of your life. Worship not in ceremony only, but in sincerity of heart.

In biblical times, when the priest entered the Holy of Holies, he would light a fire on the altar. As the flames ignited, the priest raised his hands in the air, rising with the smoke. This signified that the fire on the altar of the priest's heart still burned passionately for God.

Does your heart burn with desire for intimacy with your Creator? You don't need to be shy. Tell him everything on your mind and in your heart. Come boldly to the relationship with him. Hebrews 4:16 tells us to "draw near with confidence to the throne of grace, so that we may receive mercy and find grace to help in time of need."

Significant Ceremonies

Women love symbolism. Before marriage, some girls wear purity rings to signify that true love waits. After the wedding, our gold bands and diamonds represent our husbands' unending love for us. The anniversary, celebrated with dinner, flowers, and sometimes a second honeymoon, symbolizes that day long ago when we pledged ourselves to our mates.

Years ago, our family was looking for a symbolic Christmas tradition. We met a Jewish grandmother who taught us about Hanukkah. To our usual holiday celebration, we added several aspects of the Festival of Lights, including the lighting of the menorah, the seven- or nine-candled lampstand of the holiday. Annually, as each family member lights his or her candle, each offers up a prayer to God for the new year. We use that time to share our hearts, our dreams, and our hopes for the future; and each son or daughter receives a blessing from Mom and Dad. It's a special time!

I (Cynthia) also wanted a symbolic ceremony for my personal prayer time. So many faiths—Jewish, Catholic, Greek Orthodox, and others—use candles symbolically in their ceremonies. We have lost some traditions in the evangelical church. Less ritual can be a good thing, but we miss out on other aspects.

So I began to ask God for a smaller menorah, this one with seven candle cups, the middle higher than the rest to hold the *shammash*, or servant candle. We have seven members in our immediate family, so I figured I would use the menorah occasionally when I pray for our family. God worked a minor miracle, and I received two large brass menorahs that had served in a New York synagogue.

Though I don't use the menorah daily or as a ritual (just when the mood strikes), I have found that it enhances my worship. It's like having my own private dedication service.

First I light the shammash candle, which to me represents Jesus, who came to serve, and reminds me to show my love for my family through serving them. I claim the shammash as my own and light it first. In so many ways, the godly mother is the flame that lights faith in the hearts of her children. I remember this as my flame begins to burn. I ask for forgiveness, wisdom, and grace, dedicating myself to the Lord. Bible in hand, I pray Scripture back to him.

Then I light the candles representing each family member, pray specifically for each person, and dedicate them individually to the Lord. Sometimes I jot down anything the Holy Spirit brings to mind. After the lighting and prayers, I meditate on the glow of the candles. I pray that passion for God will burn in my heart and in the hearts of my children, so that they might know and love the Savior and always obey, serve, and glorify him. I want them to enjoy true worship of the Lord. Our lives flame up as a witness to the world. Godly families illuminate dark neighborhoods with the light and love of Jesus Christ. Finally, I dedicate our family for this purpose, perhaps with a song, always with a prayer.

We share these personal traditions, not necessarily to recommend them—these are dedications that God has given to us individually. Rather, we offer the ideas to you merely to free you up in your prayer life. You can be as creative as you like in your worship and prayer times. The King of Kings and Lord of Lords is worthy to receive our honor and glory. He is pleased by our sacrifices of praise and worship. Our prayers are one way to worship our Lord. And sometimes prayer is the only means left to us for spiritual service.

Saving the Best for Last

When Robin Finley was diagnosed with advanced non-Hodgkin's lymphoma, she determined to make each remaining day count for the Lord. Robin soon busied herself with a Romanian orphan project. Our friend purchased hundreds of copies of the Gospel of John to send to the children. She loved shopping for little clothes and toys to mail to them. Robin relished her favorite task of chauffeuring missionaries who were home on furlough. She'd drive them to restaurants, malls, and entertainment attractions in southern California, enjoying the Christian fellowship.

"I feel as if I've just begun to live," Robin once enthusiastically shared with us.

Soon, tumors on Robin's spine took the use of her legs. From her sickbed, Robin decided on a new enterprise. After cutting out hundreds of Bible flannelgraph sets, she shipped them to needy missionaries around the world. Robin also designed numerous gospel posters and tracts for them.

When paralysis hit Robin's hands, she questioned the Lord. Why had he taken away this one last avenue of service? Her missionary projects had given her purpose and meaning as she spread the gospel. *But wait a minute,* she thought. *Wasn't there one other way she could serve her Lord, even now?*

Robin explained, "When I had the use of my feet, I could go places for the Lord. Then I lost my legs. But I still had the use of my hands. I could make things for the Lord. Then I lost my hands . . . but, praise God, I still have my mind! Now I can pray to the Lord. He is so good!"

Robin's prayer ministry wrapped the world in its embrace. She developed a comprehensive plan, including not only everyone she knew, but also missionaries she knew in name only in nearly every country. Robin trusted that God knew each individual personally and would meet every need.

Robin's funeral testified through word and song how God used her life to bless others. Eternity alone will reveal the effect that she had on the world in advancing God's kingdom. Robin touched everyone who knew her with the sweet fragrance of her Savior. And she offered up to him the incense of a worshipful prayer life.

Like Hannah of old, you can draw God's greatest gifts to yourself and your world by praying to him with all of your heart. James wrote, "You do not have because you do not ask" (James 4:2). Don't be afraid to bring your needs and even your desires to your heavenly Father. He owns the wealth of the universe and is waiting to pour the bounty of heaven into your lap. According to Ephesians 1:3, you've already been offered "every spiritual blessing in the heavenly places in Christ." Prayer is the key that unlocks this treasure chest of blessing, opening it up for you and your family to enjoy.

9

Dressing for (Spiritual) Success

It's been said that the only time fashion matters is when you are out of it! Funny as that may be, we don't think it's completely true. Women of all ages seem to care about fashion. In a recent survey, 83 percent of women said they love to shop. Their number one purchase? Clothes. We ladies have a natural affinity for attractive attire.

Remember the profound truth gleaned from chapter 1: From Creation on, females have always been fashionable. And it was probably Eve's sorry idea to stitch up that first little fig-leaf tankini. She discovered pronto that God disapproved of her do-it-yourself, one-size-fits-all, unisex clothing. That was a huge mistake. But we women don't have to apologize for loving beautiful things: clothes, homes, and possessions. We have been made in God's image (Gen. 1:26–27), and God loves beauty.

Think of the grandeur of creation. Purple mountains rising from golden fields of grain. The deep-blue sea. Green meadows sprinkled with bright bits of yellow, pink, and periwinkle wildflowers. Brown bears, red foxes, orange-beaked toucans, and silvery fish. The creation is truly wonderful, isn't it? But what if the Lord had created everything in black and white? Wouldn't life be boring? For example, now that you've seen color television, would you be satisfied watching all your movies in black and white? None of us would be happy with a gray world filled with colorless people—and neither would our Creator.

> "We all wear fashionable hats. But if the Holy Spirit was allowed to genuinely, fully work in our churches, we'd all be wearing crash helmets."
>
> —author Annie Dillard

The Lord loves creative beauty, as evidenced by his specific requirements for various buildings and other constructions in Scripture. But since we are talking clothes here, think about the high priest's garments. Exodus 28 tells us that the finest materials were used to create his clothes: expensive linen in gold, purple, scarlet, and blue decorated with bright embroidery and studded with jewels like rubies, topaz, emeralds, sapphires, and diamonds. Or consider Proverbs 31, which describes an admirable woman's clothing—purple fine linen—and the scarlet wardrobe that she dressed her household in. These were colors of royalty. Other Scriptures speak of the splendor of Queen Esther and King Solomon and their royal garments.

God understands that people need nice clothes to fit into this world. And in our culture, wearing appropriate clothing can determine how you are viewed by peers, family, and coworkers.

In this chapter, we'll give you the three simple guidelines of our "dress for success" strategy: Know your colors. Know your body type. Know your personal style.

Color Me Beautiful

In college, before I (Cynthia) graduated into the beauty industry, I discovered a book by Carole Jackson called *Color Me Beautiful*. The concept of personalizing my wardrobe with color changed my look and my outlook! I discovered a wide range of hues that best enhanced my complexion and hair coloring. I applied these rules to my makeup and clothing, and wow, what a difference! I went from drab to striking—and so can you! For thirty years I have used these principles in client makeovers. The results are dramatic, thrilling the recipients. Let us briefly explain Carole's system for you.

Color Me Beautiful divides women into four color categories: winter, summer, autumn, and spring. A woman's skin tone determines whether she is in a cool (winter, summer) or a warm (autumn, spring) category. Cool complexions (no matter how dark) have blue undertones in their skin, while warm complexions have golden undertones. Look at your wrist held against a stark white paper. Does it look more blue or golden? If you have a hard time deciding, try the colors for each season around your neck, next to your face, and see which ones brighten your complexion. Each season has shades that bring out the individual's personal coloring.

The Winter woman has blue or blue-pink undertones to her skin and usually dark hair, ranging from light brown to black (and older women often have salt-and-pepper or gray hair). Winter eyes are most often a deep color of brown, hazel, gray-blue, gray-green, or dark blue. Famous Winters include Elizabeth Taylor, Cher, Jaclyn Smith, Catherine Zeta-Jones, and Oprah.

Winter's best colors are primary colors—true red, blue-red, true green, emerald green, true blue, royal blue, peacock blue, navy, royal purple, hot pinks (in brighter and deeper shades), burgundy, hospital-white, true gray, and black. The only pastels that bring out Winter's best are the palest shades of blue, pink, lavender, and green. Opt for solid colors in outfits, unless the print is bold. Never wear orange, gold, rust, peach, orange-reds, yellow-greens, beiges, or browns. Avoid dull shades; the Winter should strive to look *striking*. And she will be, when she polishes her look with her new color palette!

The Summer gal also has a complexion with blue undertones and most often some pink too. A tanned Summer may look sallow, but check an area that doesn't see the sun. Summers are usually blonde (from towhead to dark ash) as children, and often grow darker as they mature. Summers' hair coloring can range from blonde to dark ash brown, but her look is paler than a Winter. Eyes are usually blue, green, aqua, light hazel, or brown. Celebrity Summers include Princess Grace of Monaco, Cheryl Tiegs, Caroline Kennedy, Michelle Pfeiffer, and Diane Sawyer.

Summer's best colors are pastels with a blue undertone. For instance, your pinks should be true pink, not peach or salmon. Your greens should have a touch of blue, not yellow. Rosy beige or browns, gray, soft navy (never black, which is too overpowering), all shades of blue-green, all shades of blue-pink, rose, lavender, orchid, mauve, plum, burgundy, blue-red, and soft white look great on you. Avoid black, hospital-white, gold, orange, yellow-greens, or any color with yellow undertones. Opt for a *soft* look, very feminine and delicate. Use the brighter shades in your palette as splashes of color. You'll be a smash at your next big event!

The Autumn woman has a golden undertone in her skin, even when she's blushing. She can be fair with ivory skin; a redhead, often including the freckles that come with it; or a brunette with golden skin in all shades. Natural hair coloring might be red, brunette (with gold or red highlights), and occasionally black on the darker women. Most Autumns have brown or green eyes, usually with gold or brown flecks. Once in a while, an Autumn may have turquoise or aqua eyes, but never sky-blue or navy eyes. Autumns you know are Carol Burnett, Vanessa Redgrave, Katharine Hepburn, and Sara Ferguson (the Duchess of York).

Autumn's best colors are warm beiges in all tones, dark chocolate and other browns including camel and bronze, gold, yellow-gold, pumpkin, mustard, oranges, peach, salmon, rust, orange-red, yellow-green, jade, forest green, turquoise, teal, deep periwinkle. Avoid black, pinks, navy, gray, blue-red, and any other colors with blue undertones. Warmer, brighter colors look best on you, and your golden glow will warm up the room when you're dressed in your best!

The Spring lady also has a golden undertone to her skin. Often, her "peaches and cream" complexion will be the envy of her peers. Other Springs have freckles, and most have rosy cheeks. She's also the girl with the golden glow, but with less intensity than an Autumn. Her hair is golden blonde or brown, strawberry blonde, or candy red. (If you are light and your hair is ash, this is not you. See Summer above.) Some Springs have dark hair—many times hair that has darkened with age. Blue, green, or aqua are the most common eye colors for a Spring. When she has brown or hazel, golden flecks are also present. Famous Springs include Julie Andrews, Debbie Reynolds, Marilyn Monroe, and Suzanne Somers.

Spring's best colors are ivory (instead of white), warm beiges, browns from golden tan to chocolate, gold, golden yellow, yellow-gray, light navy, aqua, turquoise, light true blue, periwinkle, bright violet, peach, apricot, salmon, coral, peachy pinks, light orange, orange-red. The very fair Spring should use brighter colors as accents. All Springs should avoid black (except in prints), pure white, dark, dull colors, and all hues with blue undertones. The Spring look is *alive* with color, just like the season it represents.

Once you know your "colors," life not only becomes more exciting but also easier. For example, I (Cynthia) can go into a dress shop and head straight to my colors, avoiding shades that aren't good for me. I also avoid an hour of searching through the racks. To the shop owner's amazement, I have bought business suits in five minutes!

Comfort Rules

"I base most of my fashion taste on what doesn't itch."

—Gilda Radner

In addition, when you know your colors, the clothes in your closet coordinate, allowing you many more outfit possibilities to choose from. And you always feel assured that you look your best. In my business over the years, I have done color analysis for hundreds of women and has witnessed firsthand the astounding difference it has made in their appearance and confidence.

Body Beautiful

You may have noticed, bodies come in every size and shape under the sun. God certainly is creative! And depending on how we maintain the body he's given us, curves can be added or taken away. For the purpose of knowing your own body type and dressing appropriately, we use these classic figure categories:

1. Upside-down Triangle. This body has wide shoulders and upper body, narrow hips and thighs.
2. Rectangle. No matter how heavy or thin, this body is proportioned equally up and down, equal in shoulders and hips, with little or no indention at the waist.

Charity Chats

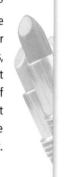

With yellow-toned skin and golden blonde hair, I am a Spring. I have seen that wearing the right colors really does make a difference. Whenever I wear my best colors—turquoise, periwinkle, or salmon—my skin glows, my eyes are brighter, and people rave about how great I look! It's almost like magic! Whenever I am doing a fashion shoot and am given a choice of several outfits, I know exactly what will look best without having to give it much thought. Many times my photographs will be chosen simply because I have learned to use color (in clothes and makeup) to bring out my best. You can learn these tricks too to become your radiant best!

3. Curvy Rectangle. Same as above, with slight indention at waist and curves at hips.
4. Pear. This body has hips and thighs that are wider than shoulders. The shape can be rounded or angular, but most of the weight is carried in the bottom half.
5. Hourglass. This body with the figure-eight shape has a bustline balanced by its hips and a narrower waist.
6. Round. This soft body carries its weight around the middle. Bustline and hips are more evenly proportioned than the pear.

What category do you fall into? Stand in front of a mirror nude or wearing undergarments or a swimsuit. Which category seems to fit your body? Next, take your measurements: shoulders, bust, waist, hips, and thighs. You can record all of this info in your "New You" Notebook. Then dress accordingly. To discover the clothes that will work best for your shape, match your type below.

- *Upside-down Triangle.* You have a dramatic appearance, with your broad shoulders and sleek lines. Be careful not to overdo with shoulder pads, puffed sleeves, and other details that further accentuate your shoulders. You can interrupt the strong vertical line with V necklines or longer necklaces. But do go with your natural shape—it's very popular. If you are big-busted, avoid cropped or bolero jackets. Choose hip-length jackets in solid fabrics (prints are too busy) over a fitted straight skirt or tapered slacks. Dresses that taper toward the knees are also striking on this figure.

- *Rectangle, Curvy Rectangle.* This body type can wear fitted dresses made of knits, jersey, silks, and other clingy fabrics. Sheath dresses, with their straight-up-and-down lines, camouflage the lack of a waist. Waisted dresses only make the waistline appear thicker, as do A-shaped dresses and skirts. A nice look is a dark skirt or slacks with a matching blouse, a belt with an eye-catching buckle, and a jacket, unbuttoned, that skims over everything.

- *Pear.* Shoulder pads in jackets and dresses help to balance your shoulders and hips. You can also use puffed sleeves, detailed necklines, wide collars, scarves, and jewelry to draw the eye toward the upper half of your body. No details at the hips, please. Colorful, interesting tops layered over dark bottoms balance your body. Avoid small, tight tops that will only make you look bigger on the bottom. The same goes for full, gathered skirts (thank heavens they went out with the pioneers). Your pants should fit well but not too tight. A jacket that skims over hips, ending just below them, is especially nice on this figure.

- *Hourglass.* This body type can show off her tiny waist in waisted and gathered designs. She can further accentuate her waist with eye-catching belts. This woman looks attractive in soft, feminine designs. Avoid stripes or plaids. Rectangle-shaped outfits hide your best feature, as do dresses that are flared from the bustline.

- *Round.* The round figure doesn't want to draw attention to her middle. And don't wear anything too baggy or too tight—this will only make you look heavier. Select clothing with long, lean lines, such as tunics over leggings, long jackets fitted with shoulder pads, dresses with dropped waistlines, blouses that hang just below the hips. Vertical lines slenderize. Draw the eye to your face with decorative collars, necklines, and jewelry.

Those clothes you see advertised in magazines look so perfect on the model, but believe me, they don't look that way in real life. Those clothes are pinned, clamped, and sewn into an exact fit. Our friend, supermodel Kim Alexis, laughs when she talks about the "illusion" of a model's perfect body. One time, she explains, her fanny was too big for a particular outfit so the photographers cut the behind out of her pants to give more room. She walked the streets of New York during the photo shoot with her bare fanny flashing behind her!

A Style All Your Own

More than anything, teens fight for the freedom to express their individuality. We've all gone through it. We shouldn't give it up now. We express who we are through the clothing we choose to wear. Business-minded, comfort-minded, trendy, feminine, sensual, zany, outdoorsy, young at heart—whatever our personality, whatever our mood of the moment, our clothes communicate. Make sure the message is yours and not a magazine's or a friend's. Analyze the style categories below to see what appeals to you:

Natural

Also dubbed the outdoorsy type, the natural gal wants to look great in an understated way. She loves the colors of nature (the four color seasons each have some of these) and fits in with the outside world. Her look is casual—nothing too fussy or dramatic.

Wear the natural tones in your season's color palette, adding a splash of color here and there in your brighter shades for interest. Opt for a layered look: sweaters and turtlenecks, vests, relaxed jackets over slacks or jeans. You appreciate fabrics with texture, like tweeds, corduroy, knits, even wool. Boots or loafers complete your outfit well.

Hair should be easy-care, something short and sleek. If long, wear it up in a topknot or casually pulled back. If permed, your curls should look like you were born with them. Don't overdo cosmetics. Your face should complete your natural look from head to toe.

Classic

The classic woman's clothes are tasteful and refined. They have a timeless quality about them. If you are a classic, your outfits fit nicely and adapt comfortably into any part of your day—shopping, business, or an evening out.

Your wardrobe should be built on the neutrals in your color palette (black, navy, or gray—Winter and Summer; brown, camel, and tan—Autumn and Spring). Choose your jackets, skirts, and slacks in these colors. Use your season's other tones in blouses and sweaters to complement (and contrast with) these. Shop for up-to-date clothing with a classy look. Don't give in to the temptation to buy something overly trendy. Pumps, classic or open-toed, go with just about everything in your wardrobe.

Keep your hair shoulder length or shorter in an unfussy style. If long, blunt the cut ends and avoid curl. Your makeup should reflect your sophistication—a face full of well-chosen cosmetics, but never flashy.

Romantic

For the romantic, the female in you is just bursting to get out! You show this in the way you dress, always very soft and feminine. You love flowing fabrics and styles. Color appeals to you, especially feminine colors like pink, red, lavenders, corals. You take time to find the perfect jewelry, with attention to every detail from hairstyle to shoes.

Dresses, long or short, with gathers, full sleeves, and flowing skirts make you feel especially feminine. Soft blouses with skirts are versatile additions to your wardrobe. You like sweaters and shawls better than buttoned up jackets. Your shoes are lacy sandals or high heels that make you feel womanly.

The romantic loves curl in her hair. Your face should complement your clothing, with lots of girlish color.

Trendy

The trendy woman knows style and is not afraid to wear it. She uses bold color (in her palette) to make her fashion statement. Her aim is high drama. When she enters the room, heads turn.

Wear oversized jackets in a striking color and slim, neutral pants or skirt. A fitted dress in a bold color is a must in this woman's wardrobe. Your shoes should also make a statement—for instance, strappy high heels under a long, lean, red jumpsuit!

Hair looks best when short or pulled back. Use color on your face to complement your outfits.

Individualist

I (Cynthia) made up this category. It covers the woman who likes all the other styles and can't figure out who she is. That's me! I enjoy being classic at times, so I wear a fitted black linen dress with wide collar and covered buttons down the front. At my son's football games, I'm all natural. Blue sweater and blue jeans over loafers. When I go out with my husband (depending on the mood I want to set), I might wear a long, flowing, feminine dress with lacy sandals and soft perfume. At a speaking engagement, my striking red suit exudes confidence (and hopefully bolsters my nerves!).

The main rule for the individualist is to have fun! You can be as creative as you want. Women who choose this style category have wild imaginations anyway—the sky's the limit on what they will come up with to wear. This girl is the one who wears a cropped sweater, a short, pleated skirt, colored tights, and combat boots. Have you seen her uptown? Well, she's the individualist! (In that case, I guess that I'm a conservative individualist.)

You can integrate the categories into any combinations you want. Wear something trendy over something feminine; something classy will combine with something outdoorsy —just try it. Remember, though, you'll look your best if you stay in your color palette (at least near your face).

You can also be creative with your face and hair. Play up one feature; understate the rest. For instance, pale skin, soft eyes, and bold, red lips. Or try bright color on both your hair and features.

A Christian Clotheshorse?

Now that you know your colors, body type, and personal style, you can head to the mall, right? Give us a minute more.

Before you hop into the car, we have a few more things to consider as Christian women. On the one hand, God understands our need for and love of beautiful clothes. On the other, he desires that our priorities stay right and that we obey several guidelines for appropriate attire.

American Heritage Dictionary

Clotheshorse (kloz hors):

1. A person excessively concerned with dress.

In Matthew 6:25, 28–30, 32–33, Jesus puts the brakes on our feverish race to Macy's sales. He said,

"Do not be worried about your life . . . as to what you will put on. Is not life more than food, and the body more than clothing? . . . Why are you worried about clothing? Observe how the lilies of the field grow; they do not toil nor do they spin, yet I say to you that not even Solomon in all his glory clothed himself like one of these. But if God so clothes the grass of the field, which is alive today and tomorrow is thrown into the furnace, will He not much more clothe you? You of little faith! . . . For the Gentiles [nonbelievers] eagerly seek all these things; for your heavenly Father knows that you need all these things. But seek first His kingdom and His righteousness, and all these things will be added to you."

Keep a balance in this area too, Jesus counsels. We can appreciate and even desire a stylish wardrobe, but we must not go overboard. As godly women, we shouldn't be known as a clotheshorse or fashion trendsetter. Our emphasis shouldn't be on our clothes, or who makes them, or how much they cost, or what size they are. Instead, we should emphasize our good works and be "famous" for them.

I want women to adorn themselves with proper clothing, *modestly* and *discreetly,* not with braided hair and gold or pearls or costly garments, but rather by means of good works, as is proper to women making a claim to godliness.

1 Timothy 2:9–10, emphasis ours

Do you claim to be a Christian? Then let your adornment be the acts by which you serve Christ and others, rather than fancy clothes, jewelry, hairstyles, and cosmetics. Beautiful clothes shouldn't be our number one priority—a beautiful spirit should. Our love affair should be with Christ, not our closet.

We do have to clothe ourselves, however. A Christian can't run around naked! As we finish this chapter, we will outline "proper clothing," as it's called in Scripture, while maintaining a balance in this delicate area. Then we'll offer some suggestions on acquiring a wardrobe that beautifully expresses who you are in Christ.

God's Word gives us very few rules regarding our wardrobes. We actually have quite a bit of freedom within the boundaries of limited scriptural guidelines. We are free to represent our personalities, personal tastes, and style in our dress. Because of this, we must be careful in our churches about judging each other by our clothing and looks.

Once, some church ladies came to Dr. McGee to complain about a lady evangelist who was visiting their town.

"Tsk! Tsk!" they gossiped. "She wears makeup."

"Yes, and she needs it!" was McGee's short quip. A good farm boy himself, he knew if the barn needs painting, paint it.

These church ladies would have been more godly to notice the evangelist's spirit. God is always looking to the heart of the person, and we should train ourselves to do that too.

Rules to Dress By

First Timothy includes two important fashion rules.

Rule Number One: Dress Modestly

Modesty is an important issue, especially in the age we live in. There's an aspect to modesty that can be cultural. For instance, what is decent dress in an African tribe would not be considered moral dressing here in the United States. (Well, on second thought, maybe it would!) What is modest today, say, dresses that fall to midcalf, would not have been proper in the 1800s or in Arab nations today where Muslim women have to cover even their faces. During Civil War days, mirrors were used to reveal immodest blind spots. Wealthy Southerners positioned gilded, full-length mirrors in their parlors and drawing rooms, and young ladies of social status would continually stand before the mirrors to check their hemlines. If even a slight bit of ankle was showing—and a young man noticed—he could go to her father and ask for her hand in marriage. Depending on the young man, this might be where the idea of miniskirts came from!

We think a good rule for modesty is to cover parts of the body that can cause lust in another person. A well-turned ankle is no longer reason for heavy breathing. But a shapely upper thigh, cleavage, or navels could bring on improper fantasies. Best to keep those areas covered.

As Christian women, we need to set a standard, show the world that we can dress modestly but fashionably. Fashion is even more important as we age. The younger woman can get by with a youthful glow. But the older woman retains her attractiveness by wearing coordinated clothing, hairstyle, and makeup, tastefully appropriate and in current styles. She dates herself when she dresses in styles popular twenty years ago (or more), whether it's hair, cosmetics, or clothes.

As mothers, we need to teach our daughters to dress chastely. At a young age, begin to reinforce this concept. Even if "all the

Cynthia Shares

Here's another angle to the controversy. Seventeen-year-old Jessica grew up in a large family with a certain philosophical persuasion. An important rule was that the females of the family always wore long-sleeved blouses and long skirts. Even when the girls played on their soccer team, they competed in their ankle-length skirts, track shoes underneath. One day, as I drove Jessica somewhere, we launched into a discussion about how believers should dress. Jessica was wearing her usual blouse and long skirt. We talked about why her church believed women should all dress that way. Of course, modesty was an issue.

I said, "Jessica, I suppose you think what I'm wearing is immodest."

"Yes, I do," she quickly replied. "Your slacks are tight, and your outfit looks like something a man would wear."

I was wearing jeans (yes, tight . . . okay, so I'd put on ten pounds!) and a very pretty pink blouse. I couldn't help but laugh at the thought of a man wearing my outfit.

Jessica continued, "Besides, Mrs. Allen, if we don't dress this way, how will the world know we are Christians?"

I immediately answered, "By our love, Jessica. Jesus said in John 13: 35, 'By this all men will know that you are My disciples, if you have love for one another.'"

other girls are wearing it," insist that your family attire themselves in styles that are pleasing to God. Bottom line. (No pun intended, but especially bottom line!) If your girls are fashion-minded, this can result in many battles, but don't become "weary in well-doing." Hang tough. They finally mature and end up dressing like Christian women should.

As daughters grow older, it helps to teach them scriptural truths so they know the "why" of the rule. They should not dress in a manner that incites a man to lust, because it could be dangerous for themselves and spiritually harmful for the man. We realize that some men are excited by just about anything, but that's their problem. As Christian women, we must remember that we will answer to God for our actions, and we want to be blameless before him. Sometimes younger women are ignorant of the emotional and sexual makeup of men. Mothers can delicately explain that men are more visual than women. They respond to outside stimuli differently than women do. We can still be beautiful women who glorify God even with something as mundane as our clothing.

Our wardrobe sends out a message into the world—a statement about our values, our moral standards, our intentions. Susan Brownmiller (author of *Femininity*) once asked, "Who said that clothes make a statement? What an understatement that was. Clothes never shut up!"

It's possible to send the message that Jesus Christ has cleaned up your life without looking like the schoolmarm on *Little House on the Prairie*. And it's possible to be stylish and attractive without wearing something too revealing.

Sometimes the clothes we wear say, "I'm successful. I will do a good job for your company." Other times it's, "I'm comfortable, and I don't care how I look." Then there's the opposite: "I'm hot. Look at me!" Or, "I know I'm not wearing much, but it's hot out here!"

Dressing immodestly puts out the wrong message for a godly woman. It says, "I'm a sexpot. All eyes on me." Instead, we want our choice of clothing to say, "I respect myself and want to be treated with respect. And more importantly, I respect God." A woman like this is not only Christlike but classy too.

We are to be "peculiar people," not because we look peculiar, but because our clean lives, good deeds, and sacrificial love are not of this world. "They are so nice/loving/honest, they're almost weird!" should be an nonbeliever's opinion of us. That's

> We really should come across as weird to the unbelieving world. Here is the American Heritage Dictionary's definition of *weird*:
>
> - Of, relating to, or suggestive of the . . . supernatural.
> - Of a strikingly odd or unusual character; strange.
>
> Let's strive for these definitions! Supernatural . . . unusual character . . . living godly lives through God's power.

how we are to stand out—not by the odd clothing we put on. Others are to be attracted to our genuinely sweet spirits and wonder what we've got that they don't. Sexy dressing or odd getups will only turn them off and turn them away.

Rule Number Two: Dress Discreetly

This concept goes hand-in-hand with modesty. But it also means something more. *Discreet* adds the feeling of not calling attention to. Have you known someone who wears clothes to call attention to herself? Our family used to occasionally turn on the television program *The Nanny* just to see what outrageous outfits Fran Drescher was wearing. Definitely not discreet, this nanny's clothes screamed for attention!

How does this apply to the Christian woman? Before your church service begins, do you walk down the aisle (a) in search of a seat; (b) to greet other worshipers; or (c) to allow the congregation to view your latest spectacular outfit? Ouch! That hurts, doesn't it? Remember the adage, clothes make the man. Well, they don't make the Christian woman. The body of believers should be attracted to the heart of the woman, not to the flashy attire she has on.

No matter what style she loves—natural, classic, romantic, trendy, or individualistic—the discreet woman always dresses in a feminine manner. The Bible talks about men dressing as men. This applies to women as well. God made us feminine creatures, and he wants us to dress that way.

Another discretionary detail is to always call attention to your face, not other areas of your body. As we have said, your eyes are the windows to your soul. You want people to be attracted to your soul and, in the process, come to know the Savior who resides there. Also, you want people to be drawn to your smile. Even non-Christians warm up to a genuine, welcoming smile.

It's important to dress appropriately as a Christian. We shouldn't dress for pretension. Some dress in their finery to show off; others dress in rags to make a rebellious statement. Either one is wrong. Remember, people look at the dress, but God looks at the heart. We must remember we have been bought with a price—the precious blood of Jesus. Then we'll glorify God with our bodies, including what we put on. We should dress in keeping with what God wants to accomplish with our lives.

A Scriptural Fashion Show

How many of you like to be stylish? Want to know what the hottest fashion is? It depends where you're going. At a funeral, black is classic. To a garden party, wear flowered chintz. A tank top and sarong at a beach barbecue. A Vera Wang original to the Oscars. If you're on your way to heaven, you'll want to know what's in style. Up there, anybody who's anybody will be wearing white. *People* magazine offers its celebrity "best-dressed list" every year. In Revelation 3:4–5, Jesus speaks of his heavenly "Who's Who," recorded for all eternity.

> But you have a few people in Sardis who have not soiled their garments; and they will walk with Me in white, for they are

worthy. He who overcomes shall thus be clothed in white garments; and I will not erase his name from the book of life, and I will confess his name before My Father, and before His angels.

You know how we watch the Oscars to see what the stars are wearing? Well, when we get to heaven, we'll look around and notice right away that the cool people—the celestial celebs—are dressed in white. We won't want to show up in anything else.

Jesus Christ's sacrifice has made us worthy to wear white. The day we receive Jesus Christ as Lord and Savior, a gorgeous white bridal gown is laid away for us in heaven. You might imagine it as an installment plan, like the way you layaway gifts for Christmas. Revelation 19:7–8 describes it:

> For the marriage of the Lamb has come and His bride has made herself ready. And it was given to her to clothe herself in fine linen, bright and clean.

How can we get these beautiful white wedding garments made of fine linen? Do all the good deeds you can in the name of Jesus Christ! Revelation 19:8 ends with, "for the fine linen is the righteous acts of the saints."

When I (Cynthia) studied the Book of Revelation inductively for two years, the above verse jumped out at me. After that, I upped my quota of good deeds. I don't know about you, but I don't want to be a streaker in heaven!

Every good deed done here on earth—done in the name of Jesus, for his glory and not for our own—is a down payment on a gorgeous white garment that we will wear for all eternity. Talk about a fashion statement! It's a "Jesus original." Although we'll wear the gown in honor, all praise will go to him on that day.

10

All That Glitters

Now that you know how to dress your body and clothe your soul, let's decorate! For your face, cosmetics are the icing on the cake, with skin care being foundational. In the same way, accessories are the icing on the fashion cake. A basic wardrobe built on the three-tiered foundation of personal color, body type, and style will see you into sensational if you dress it up with a few smart embellishments.

A little goes a long way, in both accessories and cosmetics. Simplicity adorns an outfit and a face. Take your traditional black dress. Alone, it might seem drab and ho-hum. Accented with creamy pearls, pumps, and a petite purse (black, of course), it's classy and just right. Topped with a red silk scarf pinned with a diamond and platinum brooch, and completed with red strappy heels, matching purse, and red lipstick, the same black dress becomes a head-turner.

Spend your fashion dollar wisely when it comes to accessories. But don't skimp. Wisely chosen enhancements will outlast most of the clothing pieces in your closet. Invest in the

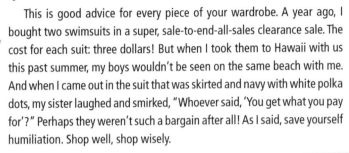

Cynthia Shares

This is good advice for every piece of your wardrobe. A year ago, I bought two swimsuits in a super, sale-to-end-all-sales clearance sale. The cost for each suit: three dollars! But when I took them to Hawaii with us this past summer, my boys wouldn't be seen on the same beach with me. And when I came out in the suit that was skirted and navy with white polka dots, my sister laughed and smirked, "Whoever said, 'You get what you pay for'?" Perhaps they weren't such a bargain after all! As I said, save yourself humiliation. Shop well, shop wisely.

best accessories that you can afford. Choose quality classic pieces that will serve you well for a long time. Trendy items can update your wardrobe, however; so if something catches your eye and it's inexpensive, take it home with you.

Accessorize Wise!

Let's see what we can do using some of our favorite accessories.

Purses

Would a girl survive without a purse? Would a family survive? My (Cynthia's) roomy purse contains my important items: wallet with undependable amounts of money; credit cards and personal info; checkbook; small notebook and assorted pens; stamps; coupons and discount punch cards for haircuts, bookstores, and pizza; hairbrush; powder; lipstick; contact solution; small hand lotion; sunglasses; Kleenex; and a pack of peppermint gum.

But it also holds my daughter's perfume and report card, my son's basketball schedule and bag of peanuts, my youngest son's three action figures with pointy parts that stick my hand when I reach in, my husband's car registration to be mailed, and that phone number he needed yesterday but I couldn't find because he wrote it on a microscopic piece of paper that fell to the bottom of the purse and has now worked its way into the lining.

Sounds like Mary Poppins, doesn't it? One of these days, this extremely stuffed shoulder bag will send me to the chiropractor. Perhaps I should invest in one of those suitcases with wheels to pull behind me! What about you? Are you the family bellhop?

Recently, I retired the catchall bag and bought a purse that has a separate zippered section on the back for license and credit cards, another for important papers and checkbook, and still more for sunglasses, a cell phone, and a holder for change. I've found that it's been worth the money in increased organization and efficiency.

Based on our experience, we've come up with this advice for buying a purse:

1. Your purse is an extension of your hand or shoulder. Choose a tastefully attractive bag.
2. A neutral shade in your color category (cool or warm) that matches your everyday shoes is best. Save bright colors for evenings or as fashion statements.
3. Your purse doesn't have to match your shoes exactly, but it should at least be the same color as your shoes.
4. Leather is costly, but it will last a long time and always has a classic look.
5. Check size in the mirror. If you are small, a very large bag may look out of proportion. The same is true for a very large woman with a very tiny purse.

6. If you have a round or pear-shaped body, don't let your purse swing at hip level. This only draws the eye to that line and widens it. (Shucks! Cynthia thought her purse hid half of her hips!)

7. For evening, clutches, envelopes, and tiny hand-bags look especially elegant. Something small. These can be beaded, metallic in silver or gold, velvet, or black leather. But these are impractical by day; they don't hold much and are easily left sitting on a counter somewhere.

8. Consider your personality when purse-shopping. An outdoorsy type would buy a bag made of natural materials like leather, straw, or alligator in earthy colors. The classic woman chooses a neutral hand-bag or clutch that matches her pumps perfectly. The romantic lady likes delicately crocheted shoulder bags in one of her pastel colors. Our trend queen opts for dramatic color in purses and shoes to make bold fashion impressions. The individualist goes creative and attention-getting—perhaps hers is that animal-print purse you thought no one would buy!

Shoes

Until recently, I (Cynthia) did not go wild when it came to shoe shopping. I have my everyday black slip-ons (which are faster when I'm running late), black evening heels (rarely worn), black business heels, red heels (rarely worn), lacy black sandals, and my jogging shoes. Except for my everyday shoes (this year's) and my exercise shoes (last year's), I've had these shoes nearly forever.

However, several months ago, a shoe store went out of business. For the price of one pair, I bought five pairs of Barbie

Doll heels in colors to match my wardrobe. They're a lot of fun but not necessary. (Plus they hurt my feet!) The general rule is: When you buy classic styles in neutral colors, the few pairs that you do have will last a long time.

1. Shop for comfort first. Your feet are the most mistreated part of your body. Give them some relief!
2. Shop for fit. Walk around the store in the shoes before buying them. Do they pinch your toes? Does the band across the top rub wrong? Is there a gap at your heel that could cause calluses? How do they feel? Buy your correct size. Get your feet measured, and don't be afraid to wear (and admit) your true size. Even supermodels do! Don't purchase shoes in the evening, because feet are often swollen after a long day.
3. If you can afford leather, go for it. It's a great investment in comfort and endurance. Avoid shoes that are obviously plastic.
4. The pump in black (cool) or beige (warm) is a must for every wardrobe and every style personality. This classic shoe will see you through the seasons, through most of your important events, and can be worn with dresses, business suits, and slacks.
5. When your shoes get scruffy looking, toss them out or give them to Goodwill. You want your look to say *polished* from head to toe.
6. Shoes that cover most of the foot are for business; lacy and strappy shoes and sandals are for dress-up occasions and evening.
7. To make your legs and ankles look longer and thinner, match hemline and stockings to shoe color; wear a one-to-two-inch heel, at least, and avoid shoes that cover the top of the foot or straps around

the ankle when wearing knee-length skirts. I (Cynthia) have a pair of black heels that have the toe and back open, but the top of the shoe covers my entire foot. When I wear these, my boys tease that I have "cankles" because it looks like my calves run right into my ankles. I now wear them only with slacks.

8. Heel height, width, and shape can date the shoe. If you don't want to replace them often, buy traditional styles.
9. Boots, especially in neutral, are a classy choice for winter. Don't allow a gap between your skirt hem and the top of your boots. Tacky!
10. Stilettos in black satin or silk are especially dressy.
11. Stockings . . . do wear them! (Bare is best with sandals, though.) Buy flesh-toned sheer hose for year-round. You can add some heavier-weight dark stockings for winter wear.
12. Shoes can also reflect your personality. The naturalist loves leather loafers; the classic, leather pumps; romantic, lacy sandals or open-backed mules; trendy, the latest style (of course); and the individualist will choose shoes in the opposite style that others expect—for instance, ruffly white sneakers with her wedding dress, shades of *Father of the Bride*!

Belts and Scarves

Belts and scarves are wardrobe extenders. They can take clothes that you are bored with and give them a whole new life. Here are some tips on choosing and wearing them correctly:

1. One-inch leather belts in neutral colors are classics.
2. Coordinate your belt to the color of your shoes and purse.

3. Or add eye-catching contrast with a bright or detailed belt if you want to show off a small waist. Great for the hourglass figure!

4. Fit your belt to your body type. The long-waisted torso matches the belt to her skirt or slacks. To cut the length of her body, she can also wear a contrasting wide belt. The short-waisted torso matches her belt to her blouse or top. A belt the same color as her dress will also elongate. Belted hip-huggers give that illusion too. Avoid wide belts that cut your short torso in half. Round or pear-shaped individuals should avoid belts period.

5. An attractive ensemble includes top tucked into slacks, a belt with decorative belt buckle, and a tailored jacket over all.

6. Scarves add life to the neutral basics in your wardrobe. They also pull together unmatched pieces of clothing into workable outfits.

7. If you want to look slimmer, wear a bright scarf at your neckline. All eyes will focus there.

8. Do you love a certain dress or blouse in a shade that's bad for you? Tie a scarf around your neck in your best color. The good color near your face will bring out your complexion.

9. Whatever your personal style, you can find scarves with just the right prints and colors. Romantics will look for florals, classics like polka-dots, trendies go for bold geometrical prints, the individualist wears an antique scarf found in grandma's attic, and the naturalist hangs a cotton sweater around her shoulders in place of a scarf.

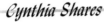

Cynthia Shares

I have one scarf that I love—a long, oblong-shaped sheer black with multicolored (including metallic silver and gold) threads running through. It goes with nearly everything in my closet. I keep it tied in a low knot, hanging on a hanger ready to go. When I want to use it, I just throw it over my black dress and run out the door.

10. Silk scarves are lovely and never go out of style. Drape one around your neck and secure with a brooch. Or, if long enough, tie one at your hips.

Glasses and Sunglasses

If you wear glasses, the days of looking like the school librarian are over. Today's glasses are important fashion accessories. Keep your frames (and prescription) updated. Choose a neutral color in your category of warm (browns, tortoiseshell, beige, or gold wire) or cool (black, navy, gray, or silver wire). Select frames in a shape opposite the shape of your face. Round faces look best with square or rectangular frames. Oblong and narrow faces need round or oval frames to widen them.

The same rules apply to sunglasses. Be sure your dark lenses have UVA and UVB protection. And always remember to wear them when outdoors.

Jewelry

Marilyn Monroe may have thought so, but she was wrong . . . diamonds are not a girl's best friend! Girls of all ages love jewelry, though, don't they? The sparkle, the shine, the incredible value of precious stones. The jewelry that women wear today can be the genuine article (fine jewelry), bridge jewelry (semiprecious stones and other natural materials), and costume jewelry (affordable imitations to enhance your wardrobe). The second and third categories are practical for most of us. Treasure any real gems you own, and use costume jewelry to add that trendy new look to your outfits.

> **"Diamonds are a girl's best friend."**
>
> —Lorelai Lee in
> *Gentlemen Prefer Blondes*

In my (Cynthia's) jewelry box I have several diamond pieces given to me by my grandparents, including my wedding set, which was my maternal grandmother's. I have two semiprecious stones, and the rest is costume jewelry that I use to spruce up my wardrobe. My favorite items are earrings, and my least favorite, rings. Because I'm always typing on the computer and playing the piano, rings get in the way.

A woman really doesn't need jewels to feel special. She's made in the image of God and loved by him—how much more special can you get than that? We can adorn ourselves with this truth and shine brightly for eternity! But we do want a few accessories to wear here. With jewelry, as with many things in life, less is more.

Your Crown Jewels

England boasts crown jewels that date back to the 1300s. Very valuable, one diamond by itself is 530 carats. If you wore a ring like that, Mr. Olympia would have to carry your hand around for you!

Don't worry if you aren't the proud owner of precious stones today. An obedient Christian has jewels laid up for her in heaven. Once I (Cynthia) did a makeover on a wealthy

Tips to Help Jewelry Work for You

1. Jewelry enhances best when in your color category. Warm complexions glow in gold; cools shimmer in silver. Everyone needs a pair of basic earrings in her metal, a simple chain in the same, and a belt buckle, if desired. Don't mix your metals, unless one particular piece is constructed with both gold and silver.

2. Your most important accessory is a watch. Punctuality graces your image better than any other adornment. Choose a timepiece in your color category: warm wears gold or brown leather; cool shines in silver or black leather.

3. Earrings can draw attention to your face if they are a bold accessory to your outfit. Color-coordinated to your eyes, they show off great features. Round earrings enhance long faces; dangling earrings add length to round faces. Ears look great adorned with jewelry. But they were made for more! Hearing God's Word is their most important function.

   "Truly, truly, I say to you, he who hears My word, and believes Him who sent Me, has eternal life, and does not come into judgment, but has passed out of death into life" (John 5:24).

   "Prove yourselves doers of the word, and not merely hearers who delude themselves " (James 1:22).

4. If you have long, lovely nails, definitely wear bracelets with sleeveless or short sleeved blouses to bring the focus to your hands.

5. A sparkling pin or brooch is a necessity to add interest to a jacket, for holding scarves, or even pinning at your waist to draw eyes there.

6. Short necklaces enhance long faces; long necklaces, even those dropping to the waist, create the illusion of a slimmer face and longer torso.

7. Use the rule of three. Three has the feeling of completion. A trinity of matching accessories works the same way. For instance, if you're wearing oval pearl earrings, also use a pearl brooch and ring. If your earrings are gold rectangles, wear a belt buckle and ring in the same shape and metal.

8. The one-hue rule: Repeat the boldest color in your outfit several times in your accessories. For instance, if you're wearing a red jacket over black slacks and shirt, add red earrings, a red belt, purse, and mules. Don't forget your red lipstick—wow, what a look! If you have a warm complexion and a more subdued personality, try wooden accessories with your camel-colored jacket and slacks. Classy!

9. Don't forget to invest in a strand of pearls. These gems are easy to wear and dress up any outfit. You can't go wrong with pearls.

client. The young blonde flashed her huge diamonds in my face and began bragging about them. I looked down at my plain little naked fingers and felt like stammering, "I . . . I . . . I have some jewels too. They're just not here. I don't want them stolen. They're in a safe-deposit box in heaven!"

> "Greater love has no one than this, that one lay down his life for his friends."
>
> —Jesus Christ, John 15:13

It's true. Do you keep a vision in your head of the day you'll stand alone before Christ? First, he'll give you your white linen gown. Designed especially for you, the dress is created by your faith in Christ and the righteous, obedient acts you've done. Then the Lord will present you with your crown jewels. He will reward you for your commitment to your marriage. Then, one by one, he'll call your children up. Jesus will reward you for your perseverance in raising your children in the Lord. He'll honor you for all the people you've witnessed to in word or deed, for all those you helped in his name.

When you have your jeweled crown in hand, you'll then kneel before Jesus and lay it at his feet. The gems actually belong to him. Without Jesus giving us everything necessary to live this life, we would have no victory.

Like we said, a girl doesn't need jewels to feel special!

Power Dressing

We talk about dressing for success in this world. What about dressing for spiritual success? Would you like some beautiful jewelry to wear for all eternity? How about gold?

> In this you greatly rejoice, even though now for a little while, if necessary, you have been distressed by various trials, that

the proof of your faith, being more precious than gold which is perishable, even though tested by fire, may be found to result in praise and glory and honor at the revelation of Jesus Christ.

1 Peter 1:6–7

Has your precious faith been tested by fire? Both of us have had our faith tested.

Our family felt relieved when 1994 was officially over. We had just been through two years of what seemed like nearly every problem under the sun. I (Cynthia) had experienced a difficult pregnancy and the near death of our fifth child. Months of caring for a newborn with a life-threatening illness plus four other children flared my chronic auto-immune problems, causing my physical collapse. Then I was hospitalized for exploratory surgery for cancer. We lost a third of our income and our house. Financial problems mounted, marriage difficulties surfaced, and friendships faded away.

Through our family's experiences, I've learned a few lessons. Tough times are guaranteed to come in life. The key issue is how people respond to them. It was such a gift that God allowed me to live to raise my children. Even more important is the gift of a growing faith that, when tested by fire, shines through like pure gold. Here are some suggestions for developing faith when times are tough.

Commit. Early in your troubles, reaffirm your commitment to God. Try listing every person and thing in your life that is important to you in a notebook, maybe even your "New You" Notebook. The Lord is big enough to take care of your concerns, isn't he? When you are tempted to worry, review your list. Commit your worries to the Lord. The beautiful woman has a mind and heart at rest.

Charity Chats

God allowed me to go through the fire—literally! In my junior year of college, I was an intern at Focus on the Family in Colorado. Before this, college life had meant dorms and everlasting slumber parties. But suddenly I had my own apartment and much unaccustomed solitude. One day I was badly burned in a kitchen fire. A stranger rushed me to the hospital. I spent months enduring painful therapy at a burn center, with the kind of treatments that were making grown men around me cry. I went through this experience alone—no family or friends were there to comfort me. The only Person I had was the Lord. For the first time in my life, I depended on him completely. Before that, I'd always depended on my family for spiritual support. I came out of that experience an independent Christian in my own right. In my "fiery" trial, God taught me who he is and what trusting him really means. My faith was strengthened, and Scripture promises that our faith is more precious than gold.

Then continue with your commitment of daily time spent in the Word and in prayer. These times with the Lord can sustain you like nothing else can.

Cling. Circumstances can get so bad that they shake even the most faithful. In those moments, cling to the Lord and to those you love with all your might. During her difficult times my mother wrote in the margin of her Bible, "Trust! Trust! Trust!" Her simple motto has encouraged me to keep hanging on, come what may.

We must surround ourselves with people who build our faith and provide hope. Negative influences pull us down at a time when we need lifting up. Think of Job's discouraging friends. Even his wife advised the poor man to "curse God and die." Develop a network of positive encouragers. With them, you can cry when you're scared and rejoice when things improve. Their support will help you to stay afloat when stormy waves threaten to engulf you.

Choose. Nothing brings more honor to the Lord than seeing his children experiencing peace, joy, and patience in the midst of tribulation. Make a conscious decision at the onset of your problems to give God praise throughout your trials. That commitment will be tested many times. But hold firm.

Count. The song counsels us to "Count your blessings—name them one by one; Count your blessings—see what God hath done."[1] When things are going great, it's hard to keep a song from our lips. But let things turn sour, and it takes an effort to find something positive to say, right? But that's when it's most glorifying to God to sing, praise, and give thanks. Scripture calls it "a sacrifice of praise." A sacrifice means giving up something, doing the hard thing, or offering up something valued to someone deemed greater. Like the widow's mite, our praise is far more valuable to God when it comes out of loss rather than abundance. Hebrews 13:15 says:

> Through Him then, let us continually offer up a sacrifice of praise to God, that is, the fruit of lips that give thanks to His name.

How can we offer this sacrifice of praise in the midst of a trial? Through Christ. Our friend Marge learned to "give thanks in all things." As the mother of eleven children, nearly all of them grown, all doing well, Marge was particularly blessed. But then tragedy struck her family: Her daughter-in-law and daughter died within months of each other, and, soon after that, her husband had a stroke. In spite of her grief, Marge desired that her response be right. She asked the Lord to give her things to be thankful for. Soon she began noticing the miracles, even the minor ones, in each situation. The list for her daughter-in-law contained eight praises; her daughter's record of praises reached seventeen. Her husband's list is growing.

"I'm not thankful that my daughters died and my husband became sick," Marge explains. "But God gives us things to be thankful for in our calamities. These thanksgiving lists were the very things that helped me not to sink under the river of grief. They kept my head above water. Even though I was going through a rough time, I could still see God working."

Marge is a beautiful testimony of a trusting spirit, a faith more precious than gold when tested by fire. She has certainly earned her heavenly crown to wear. But like us, she will lay it at the feet of Jesus. For Marge knows that it was God's grace that sustained her through great difficulty. In the midst of heartache, the Lord gave this mother the gift of a thankful heart. And for all eternity, she will give the praise and honor and glory to him.

Want some gold that won't tarnish or be taken away?

- Commit to Christ, no matter what.
- Cling to him, his promises, and to those who love his appearing.
- Choose to glorify him, come what may.
- Count your blessings, even when it's a sacrifice.
- Thank God that he's giving you the opportunity to learn to trust him more.

Jesus is laying away for you an unfading crown of glory that will be your reward for all eternity. The apostle Paul, who knew as much suffering as any man, promises in Romans 8:18 that "the sufferings of this present time are not worthy to be compared with the glory that is to be revealed to us."

Hang in there, sister. That day is worth waiting for!

Epilogue

The Finishing Touch

While dressing, most women have one last thing they do before they walk out the door. Whether it's a spritz of perfume or hairspray, a flick of a brush, or a quick glance in the mirror, it's a final ritual that says, "I'm finished. I'm just right. I'm ready to put my best face forward."

The authors want to do that just now, in these final pages. We'd like to send you off with blessings and prayer. In *The Beautiful Balance,* you have seen a concept of wholeness illustrated. To become the truly beautiful women that we all hope to be, we must balance our focus between the physical and spiritual. Our time and energies should be concentrated on developing strong relationships with Christ, on cultivating Christian character, while not neglecting the care of our physical attributes.

We've come to our final chapter—the end of the book, but not the end of our journey. To become the very best we can be, we all must keep learning, growing, and polishing up our persons, both inside and out. In their book *The Power of Focus*, authors Jack Canfield, Mark Victor Hansen, and Les Hewitt have this to say:

> People who are rich in every sense of the word understand that life is a learning experience. It never stops. Learn to constantly refine your habits. There is always another level to reach for, no matter how good you are right now. When you constantly strive to improve, you build character. You become more as a person, and you have more to offer. It's an exciting journey that ultimately leads to fulfillment and prosperity.[1]

Hopefully, you have begun to build new habits.

Exercise and proper nutrition are now a part of your life (you can find advice in *The Healthy Balance*). In a short time, you'll be rewarded for your efforts with more energy and strength and clothes that fit more loosely. And your clothes—you're beginning to build a wardrobe of clothing and accessories that complement in color, style, and fit. Your signature scent ensures that you smell as good as you look.

> **"Balance doesn't just happen. To achieve it we must first establish our priorities."**
>
> —Mary Kay Ash, founder of Mary Kay Cosmetics

You've started a hair- and skin-care program of cleansing and conditioning. You protect your skin and hair from harsh elements, including the sun. Your manicured hands and feet are being used to touch lives and spread the gospel. You are practicing makeup application and receiving the compliments that come to a woman who sparkles. And you now realize that your best accessory is your own beautiful smile!

From the top of your head down to your pedicured toenails, your hard work has paid off. Isn't it great to walk into a room and know that you look your best?

The authors have thirty-nine combined years in the beauty industry. We've seen just about everything there is to see. But one thing we are sure of: There is something physically beautiful about every woman.

My (Cynthia's) clients come to me for makeovers unhappy with their looks. As I study each woman's skin, coloring, and face, I search for the good features to emphasize. Perhaps the woman has striking blue eyes that twinkle with secret laughter. Or she may be the proud owner of the straight nose of a Grecian goddess. Creamy skin and shimmering copper hair make her a standout. Or her smile may be as contagious as Julia Roberts's. When I observe these and other assets, I am gratefully aware that God has placed his stamp of beauty on each of his feminine creatures. Every woman, even those who feel like plain Janes, has something she can thank God for!

On the other hand, I (Charity) have observed that some of the world's most beautiful women aren't satisfied with their looks. Yes, models have learned to make the most of the assets God gave them—to maintain their bodies with wise eating and exercise, to dress to flatter, to wear enhancing cosmetics correctly, to stand tall, assured of who they are.

But models are also very aware of their own flaws. They have mirrors and eyes to see the truth. In addition, they have critical photographers, makeup artists, and directors broadcasting their shortcomings. The pressure to be perfect is intense. Why do you think so many models turn to drugs and other means of escape?

Even as a Christian, I once caved under the pressure. In that moment, though, I discovered God in a powerful way that still impacts me today. I was a novice model who fell into the business when I was approached one day while shopping in a department store. The scout took my name and number, and soon I began getting calls for commercials and advertisements.

At one of these first auditions, something happened that gave me an attitude adjustment. I got the call at the last minute while out shopping and hurried over to the interview unprepared. I was wearing old blue jeans and a blah brown sweater, which didn't help my confidence! I didn't have my "zed-card" (examples of photos previously taken) or résumé.

Wearing this lack of assurance, I walked into the waiting room filled with other models—Nikki Taylor and Naomi Campbell look-alikes—all hoping to snag the job. Every pretty head turned and stared at me, giving me the "once-over" with a sneer and a huff. Their glare confirmed my worst fear: I didn't belong there. These women were stunning! At least six feet tall and all legs. (I have a glaring "defect" in the modeling world—I'm very petite, five-feet, six-inches, and small-boned. A modeling midget!) Each girl was stick-thin with huge breasts that overshadowed my miniature size 32, nearly B-cup bra!

"I don't have a chance here," I said to myself. And so I did my usual thing: began to make the rounds being friendly. I talked to each model and asked to see her portfolio, praising each photo. When it was my turn in front of the camera, I didn't take it seriously. I knew I wouldn't be chosen for the opportunity, so I joked and laughed. But in the car on the drive home, the laughing stopped. I bawled and bawled. Once home, I fell on my knees, pouring out my heart to the Lord.

"I wanted so badly to stand out today, Lord, for them to see something extraordinary, something special about me. What was I thinking? Why even try? I don't measure up. I'm nothing compared to those beautiful, flawless women. I'm hardly perfect, Lord, as you well know. What do I have to make people notice me?"

Through my tears, an inaudible voice reached my heart loud and clear.

"You have me," the Lord spoke to my heart. "I am the difference that others notice about you. It is my Spirit that draws others to you and my love that wins their hearts. I am what's special about you, Charity. I, alone, am your one true beauty."

I will never forget my Savior's words; they have changed my life forever. The truth of God's message was confirmed one week later when the call came from the casting director saying that, out of all the girls, they had chosen me.

"Why me?" I wondered aloud.

"We liked your attitude," he said. "We'd love to work with you, Charity. There's something different about you."

We know what that difference is. And so do you, dear woman of God. It's Jesus Christ, the One who is "altogether lovely." Blessings as you continue spending time with him, in his Word and in prayer. (We'll remember you; you pray for us!) It's the most important part of your day. The increased joy and peace in your life will be the evidence of this commitment. Allow your godly character to shine through as you reach out to your world with words and deeds that send a message of God's love.

And God bless you as you continue to work through this book, focusing on those areas that need improvement, both in body and soul. Fill your "New You" Notebook with the record of your progress, pictures to prove it, and dreams for your future. Clairol, the cosmetic company, once had this motto: "A beauty all your own." As you apply principles learned in *The Beautiful Balance,* you will discover the radiant beauty all your own that God created you to have.

When women become their best in body and soul, their joy, confidence, and hope spread out into the world—first, to their families, then on to their neighbors, and eventually to the ends of the earth. Try some inner and outer makeover magic, as outlined in this book, and you'll experience the beautiful balance that only the Lord Jesus can bring to a life.

Notes

Chapter 1: The Beautiful Balance

1. Karen Lee-Thorp and Cynthia Hicks, *Why Beauty Matters* (Colorado Springs: NavPress, 1997), 94.

Chapter 4: More Than Skin Deep

1. Spiros Zodhiates, ed., *The Complete Word Study Dictionary: New Testament* (Chattanooga: AMG Publishers, 1992).

Chapter 7: Hands That Walk, Feet That Talk

1. Found online at several sites with no author attributed, but attributed to Paul Ciniraj at <http://1stholistic.com/Prayer/hol_prayer_it-all-depends-ciniraj.htm>.

2. Fulton J. Sheen, quoted at <http://www.bartleby.com/63/72/4272.html>.

Chapter 10: All That Glitters

1. Johnson Oatman Jr. and Edwin O. Excell, "Count Your Blessings," in *Great Hymns of the Faith* (Grand Rapids: Zondervan, 1975), no. 370.

Epilogue

1. Jack Canfield, Mark Victor Hansen, and Les Hewitt, *The Power of Focus* (Deerfield Beach, Fla.: Health Communications, 2000), 21.

Resources

For Bible teaching:

Precept Ministries International, inductive Bible studies by Kay Arthur

1-800-763-8280 or www.precept.org

In Touch Ministries, teaching by Pastor Charles Stanley

1-800-789-1473 or www.intouch.org

Focus on the Family, teaching by Dr. James Dobson

1-800-661-9800 or www.fotf.org

Thru the Bible Ministries, teaching by Dr. J. Vernon McGee

1-800-65-BIBLE (24253) or www.ttb.org

For Scripture memorization:

Jack Van Impe Ministries, www. jvim.org

For further reading:

Why Beauty Matters by Karen Lee-Thorp and Cynthia Hicks (NavPress, 1997)

Fresh-brewed Life by Nicole Johnson (Thomas Nelson, 1999)

The Power of a Praying Woman by Stormie Omartian (Harvest House, 2003)

The Secrets of an Irresistible Woman by Michelle McKinney Hammond (Harvest House, 1998)

The Pursuit of God by A. W. Tozer (Christian Publications, 1993)

Loving God by Charles Colson (Zondervan, 1997)

More about the Authors...

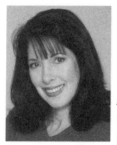

A veteran in the beauty industry since 1973, **Cynthia Culp Allen** has worked as a licensed cosmetologist and image consultant, helping women become their best through personal consultations and printed advice. She has published over six hundred articles in publications like *Focus on the Family, Brio, Guideposts,* and *Decision.* Honored with six national writing awards, the author has contributed to eight best-sellers, including *Chicken Soup for the Christian Family Soul* (Health Communications), *The Hidden Hand of God* (Guideposts), *God's Vitamin C for the Hurting Spirit* (Starburst Publishers), *Raising Them Right* (Focus on the Family), and *The Women's Devotional Bible II* (Zondervan). Her devotional series, Innerludes, published by Cumberland House, includes *Home Is Where You Hang Your Heart,* a book for mothers, and *More Encouraging Than Flowers,* a devotional for the sick and grieving. Cynthia is a popular speaker for churches, conferences, and retreats and has also been a guest on several radio and television programs.

This mother of five lives in northern California with her husband, Charles, and her three younger children. She stays busy with her writing and speaking, home schooling her children, and taking long walks in the country. Cynthia can be reached for speaking engagements and guest appearances at P.O. Box 1313, Chico, CA 95927-1313, or e-mail: cynthiaculpallen@yahoo.com.

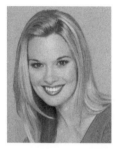

Charity Allen Winters is an established model in the fashion industry. Her print work can be found in such publications as *Sunset Magazine, Focus on the Family, Living with Teenagers, Brio, Bongos,* and *Model USA.* She is also a rising actress who is recognized in Europe as the lead host of "Liberty Television" and has also been featured on many national television shows, including *Just Shoot Me,* Disney's *So Little Time,* and MTV.

As a recording artist, she has soloed with the Los Angeles Opera Company and has made a variety of television appearances, opened for country star Charlie Daniels, and was an honored guest at a performance at the Canterbury Cathedral. After her 1999 graduation from Biola University with a B.A. in Mass Media Communications, Charity has spent recent years traveling the country as a speaker and gospel singer but loves coming home to her new husband, Kelvin, in Los Angeles. She can be contacted directly for speaking, singing, and guest appearances by e-mail: message4charity@yahoo.com, or booked through Paul Webb at Hollywood Pacific Studios, (818) 349-2093.

The
life balance
Bulletin

Are you like us—
do you love to receive mail?
Well, we'd love to send it to you!

The LifeBalance Bulletin,

our quarterly newsletter,
is packed with fresh fashion tips,
seasonal health and beauty advice,
and spiritual insights to satisfy your soul.
In addition, learn about the latest
LifeBalance products, including how to order your own

"New You" Notebook!

For a one-year subscription to
The LifeBalance Bulletin, register online at
www.lifebalanceladies.com

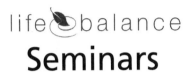

Seminars

Authors and motivational speakers Cynthia Culp Allen and Charity Allen Winters travel the country inspiring women of all ages to become their best through LifeBalance Seminars. At these life-changing conferences, women learn the art of life balance in the following areas:

The Beautiful Balance Seminar

Celebrate the power of a woman's beauty, inside and out.

The Healthy Balance Seminar

Learn the secrets for physical wellness, weight loss, and inner strength.

The Inner Balance Seminar

Rejuvenate health through the purification of body and soul.

The Beautiful Balance for Teens Seminar

Grow in the beauty of Christ together as mother and daughter.

To schedule a LifeBalance Seminar or for specific conference information, visit www.lifebalanceladies.com.

MIRACLE MAKEOVERS . . .

They can happen to you!

Continue your journey
with the latest advice for
body and soul.
Visit our website at

www.lifebalanceladies.com

where you can interact with the authors
in a question-and-answer forum,
preview new releases and LifeBalance products,
and
keep up with the LifeBalance conference
and events schedule.

We hope you'll visit us soon!

The LifeBalance Ladies,

Cynthia   Charity

Revolutionary New Skin Care Products

The LifeBalance Ladies are excited to introduce two new revolutionary skin care products—Natasha's Probiotic Daily Cleansing Preparation and Natasha's Probiotic Face Cream—produced by Natren, the world's leader in probiotics. Probiotics are good bacteria including lactobacilli like acidophilus, bifidus, and others. These protective products guard your skin's precious acid mantle and encourage cell growth and renewal.

Natasha's Probiotic Daily Cleansing Preparation exfoliates gently with crushed apricots, walnuts, and almonds, removing dead skin cells while it cleans. Hypoallergenic, it's perfect for every skin type.

Natasha's Probiotic Face Cream contains probiotics and other cutting-edge, high quality ingredients that will exfoliate, moisturize, and repair. Vitamins and botanicals add nourishment to the skin while the probiotics repair cells and condition. Cleopatra (and other beauties of the ancient world like her) knew the secrets of lactic acid, using nature's gifts to retain her legendary beauty—and you can do the same!

What people are saying about Natren skin care products:

- "Rich, yet absorbs quickly."
- "Non-greasy, in spite of the luxurious texture."
- "I never thought a moisturizer would help my acne!"
- "Doesn't leave a shine, but dries to a silky, powdery finish on my face!"

To order Natasha's skin care line, visit our web site at www.life balanceladies.com or call Natren direct at 800-992-3323 and mention the LifeBalance Ladies, Cynthia Culp Allen and Charity Allen Winters.

Coming soon . . .

The Healthy Balance for Body and Soul
The next transforming step in becoming a beautifully balanced woman. It's hard to shine when you're feeling shoddy . . . so this book offers the latest advice on nutrition, weight loss, fitness, and other important aspects of a healthy, balanced lifestyle.

Available in stores in time for your 2004 New Year's resolutions!

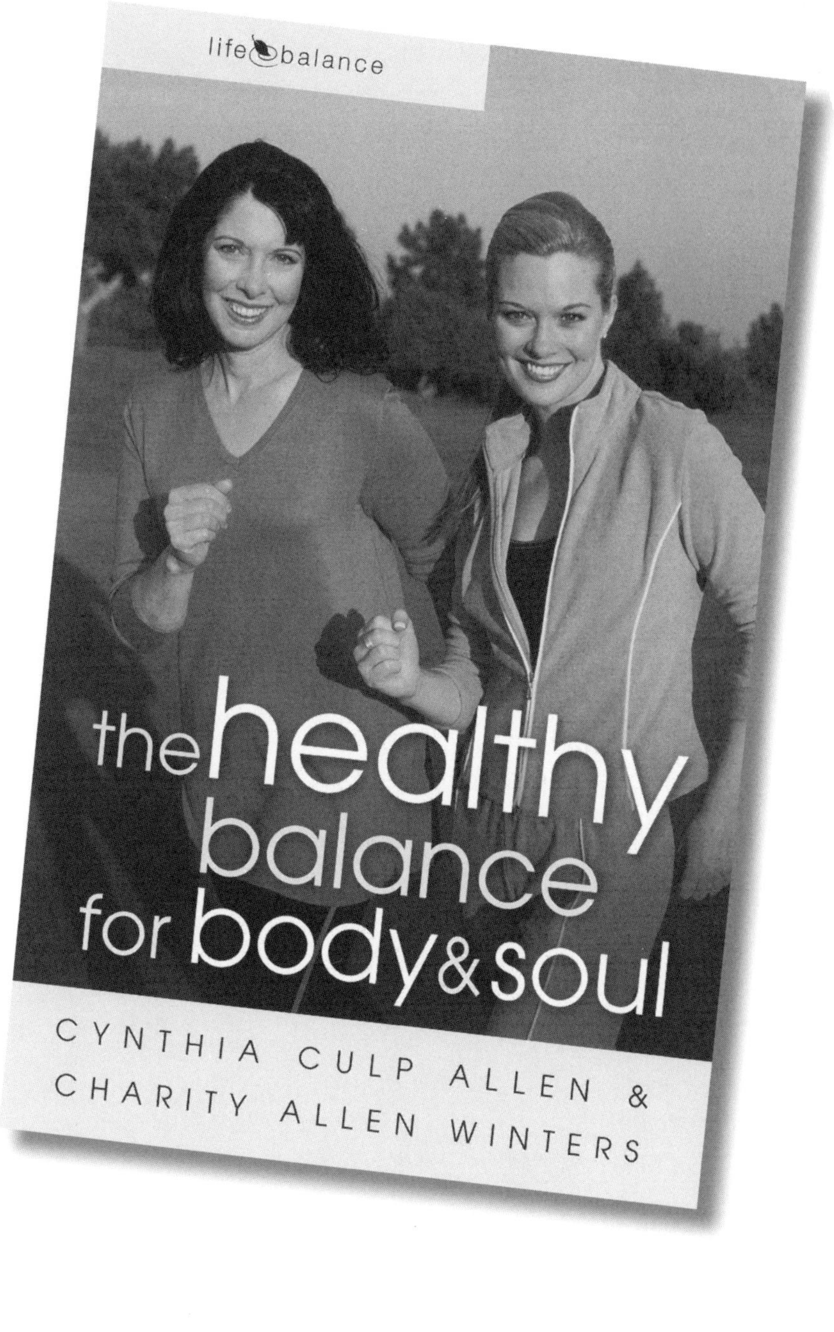
life balance
the healthy balance for body & soul
CYNTHIA CULP ALLEN &
CHARITY ALLEN WINTERS